…the kids are still playing nice together in the sandbox!

I never had any intention of writing another book
or having a second lung transplant either.

Jim Carns

Single Left Lung – September 22, 2013

Single Right Lung – August 10, 2021

FORWORD

I just received a phone call from Jim Carns, one of the most amazing people I know. He asked if I would be interested in writing a foreword for his second book about his journey through a second lung transplant, the title was undecided at the time. Yes, you heard this correctly, his second lung transplant. I knew he was writing about his experience and I could not wait to read and share it with patients and families exploring, embarking on this journey. My heart jumped and I happily said, "Wow, Jim, it would be an honor."

The exact date I met Jim Carns was Friday, August 19, 2016. He sent an email sharing his newly published book "New Mountains to Climb", and it said "Before you delete this email because you think it is Spam, please let me introduce myself. My name is Jim Carns and I belong to the IPF Support Group at the Hershey Medical Center, located in Hershey, PA. I received my "second chance" at life on September 22, 2013, at Temple University Hospital in Philadelphia where I received the left lung of an unknown donor. "From that point, I am privileged to have Jim and Karen (Jim's wonderful wife) Carns be an active and integral part of our organization, the Wescoe Foundation for Pulmonary Fibrosis.

My name is Jennifer Wescoe Singley, Executive Director of the Wescoe Foundation for Pulmonary Fibrosis. Wescoe Foundation for Pulmonary Fibrosis is a 501(c)3 non-profit organization that provides support, education, advocacy, and resources for the patients, their families, and care partners, in order to sustain the highest possible quality of life. Often patients, care partners, and families feel overwhelmed and uncertain of what the future holds while living with pulmonary fibrosis. Through our support groups, educational programs, and community awareness events, we strive every day to help the pulmonary fibrosis community navigate this serious lung disease.

Throughout the past six years, I have given Jim's book, "New Mountains to Climb" to patients we serve as well as people attending our lung transplant educational series. It has been a tremendous help for patients who are at the stages of pre-, peri-, and post-lung transplant. Jim's experience has brought levity, humor, real life, and honest experience that I know that people can learn from and relate to. I have also distributed the book to pulmonologists and other healthcare professionals to learn more about a person's experience with a lung transplant. It has proven to be effective in their practice in truly understanding the patient experience.

Jim has not only received one lung transplant but two. His strength, unwavering optimism, and honesty will continue to be a beacon of hope for many throughout their lung transplant journey. If anyone is going to help others through his life experience, it's Jim Carns. I highly recommend Jim's book as a must-read for patients, care partners, and health care professionals.

Respectfully,

Jennifer Wescoe Singley, M.Ed., NCC

Executive Director

Wescoe Foundation for Pulmonary Fibrosis

www.wescoe.org; www.paipfsupportnetwork.org

jennifer@wescoe.or

"... the kids are still playing nice in the sandbox" is the title I have chosen for the next chapter of my journey with Idiopathic Pulmonary Fibrosis that I began in 2009. I was diagnosed with this dreaded disease that claims almost 30,000 individuals each year, yet many people have never heard of Pulmonary Fibrosis.

Currently, there are more than 106,000 people in the United States on the organ transplant waiting list, with more than 1,000 of those awaiting a lung transplant.

You are probably reading this and saying to yourself, what a strange title for a new book. Well, maybe, but let me explain why it makes perfect sense to me.

I had my first single lung transplant back on September 22, 2013 and have been carrying the left lung, which I call 'Juan' in honor of my first donor. In 2019, I was diagnosed with Bronchiolitis Obliterans Syndrome, BOS for short, and in 2020 I was listed for my second single lung transplant.

Having had my second single lung transplant on August 10, 2021, I now carry a right lung, which I affectionately call 'number two' only because I do not know much about this donor.

I have two different lungs in my chest, from two different donors; the kids I refer to in the title are my lungs and my chest cavity is the sandbox. So far everything is good, and the kids are still playing nice in the sandbox! Now it makes perfect sense to you!

Introduction

According to the Scientific Registry of Transplant Recipients (SRTR), I find myself in a unique situation, and I think my story is worth sharing.

I had no intention of writing another book, and now as I think about it, I never had any intention of having a second lung transplant either.

I know what some of you might be thinking, it seems like just a short time ago I told my story about my journey with pulmonary fibrosis and my first single lung transplant. This may be true, but it has been a little more than six years. It was in December 2015 I stopped putting my thoughts about my transplant journey on paper and decided to try my hand at publishing a book about my journey. With the help of my family and friends, my book, *New Mountains to Climb* was finally published in July of 2016 and is still available on Amazon.

Here it is, the beginning of 2022, and much has changed with me since then. I won't say the eight years since my first transplant have been terrible, but for the most part it definitely has been different in many ways.

The next chapter of my journey will briefly bring us all up to date from where *New Mountains to Climb*, left off. The next chapter of my journey really begins in 2019, but first I have a big hole to fill until I get there.

Originally, I started writing *New Mountains to Climb* as a journal to share with my family, a record, if you will, of how my first transplant journey transpired, I have no plans to give a detailed account of daily activities in Section I. I will probably stray from this statement in Section II of my new book "***...the kids are still playing nice together in the sandbox!***," when I talk about my second transplant and events leading up to it.

We have a lot of real estate to cover to get us all up to date, so, let's get the next part of my journey started.

SECTION I

2015 – 2018

In SECTION I, I will not belabor you with details of every single day, but I will point out some of the more important things happening during this period of time. I will honestly say, staying active is a key part of this 6+ year journey we are on, and I tried my best to do just this. If you read my first book, *New Mountains to Climb* you will see I did not just sit around but rather stayed as active as possible.

After my first transplant in 2013, I spent time with our grandkids at Hershey Park; we spent two plus weeks in Alaska and on a cruise to Hawaii and even a river cruise in Europe. Just because I have a disease I didn't ask for; it doesn't mean I have to sit around and wait for the end to come. I refuse to let pulmonary fibrosis take control of me. I still exercise and currently go to pulmonary rehab.

One disclosure I must make is this, when I refer to "we," for the most part I will be referring to my wife/best friend Karen!

1

<u>2015</u>

I really thought it might be easy to write about the continuation of my journey by doing it month by month, but I am finding much of what I write in this section is very repetitive. This is something I am trying to avoid, so I am going to try and touch on the highlights or lowlights, whatever they may be.

Like I said in my previous book or at least tried to say, you can't live in a shell with no exposure to the world outside the little bubble we, as transplant patients, tend to live in. We went to Bethany Beach to bring in 2015 with close friends. I had some New Year resolutions I needed to make, and the beach seemed like a good place to make them. When the opportunity arises, we try to do different things to remain active and going to the beach is just one of the things we like to do.

We attended our son's military retirement ceremony and spent a few days in the Alexandria, VA area, in May; we also visited family in Kansas City, MO and West Bend, WI.

Healthwise, I have been doing great. I had appointments with Dr. Cordova, my primary transplant pulmonologist, in Philadelphia every three months or so and his team continues to be quite pleased with my recovery. The only thing they continue to do is tweak some of my medicines, and they have been doing this from day one and probably will for the rest of my life.

During this period, I continued with the proverbial three blows and go pulmonary function tests (pft's), and blood draws. I also had a colonoscopy, x-ray, ekg and a bone density scan which were part of my normal testing routines. In the grand scheme of things, all were normal and life is great.

If you read my previous book, you might remember, back in August of 2014 it was suggested I have a Sleep Apnea Study completed. I did the study in October and my doctor said we would discuss the findings at my January appointment. Dr. Cordova asked how I was doing with the c-pap machine. I honestly told him I was getting less sleep and probably was waking more often than before. He looked at his notes and said my sleep apnea is on the 'mild side." I had told him before that I didn't need to use nor want to use the machine if it wasn't helping me. Now I know this machine helps many people, but I am one patient it did not help.

 As if I haven't endured enough over the past couple of years, this month I attended a Neil Diamond concert. In honesty it wasn't bad and I enjoyed the concert. This was a combination birthday present for my wife as well as a token of my appreciation for all she has done for me since being diagnosed, the transplant, and beyond. I can't imagine what I would have done without her.

One of the more practical things we did, and this is not meant to be morbid in any sense of the imagination, but we made our final arrangements with our funeral director. Plans are done and everyone knows our wishes. We don't plan on using any of his services anytime soon.

In September we decided to start "paying it forward" for some of what we have received during our journey to date. Along with other family members, we provided a complete home-cooked meal for the guests staying at the Gift of Life

Family House in Philadelphia. This is an event we still do annually, except for 2020 when the COVID-19 pandemic got in the way. Truthfully, COVID-19 also got in our way again in 2021, but we still were able to provide a meal for the guests, even though it was not homemade. As soon as we get the green light, we will be doing it again in person.

Spending time with family and friends has been high on our list. We have been to more sporting events than I care to count, and even to a few events I don't quite understand. Birthdays and special events for family have always called for a cookout, lunch or dinner.

Participating in our monthly support groups, raising money for them and even speaking on their behalf kept me active.

I guess what I am trying to say in this part is this, health wise I have had a pretty great year, I just didn't sit around doing nothing. I did things with family, friends, church, organizations and we did things together. However, when dealing with this disease, you must stay as active as possible. Yes, I am well aware somedays it is hard to get moving and that's alright, but you must be as active as you can both pre-and post-transplant.

It would be quite easy for me to be able to fill pages with minute details of what is happening in my life. To be honest I have had twelve months of "pretty smooth sailing."

<u>2016</u>

If this year has as few health issues as last year, I will have little to discuss and I will be on our way to begin writing about next year.

I start 2016 just like I start every year. In order to bring us luck for the upcoming year, our family has a pork and sauerkraut dinner. This is an old Pennsylvania Dutch tradition which supposedly brings you luck throughout the upcoming year.

Karen, my wife, had a total knee replacement so our roles were reversed for a few weeks; I became the caregiver and she was the patient. I got a very small taste of what it was to be a caregiver. I believe her job of being a caregiver to me was probably much more difficult.

Let's talk a little bit about what was happening with me this year. Although in the grand scheme of things, this year could have been worse, but it wasn't. I am still here and kicking.

I had my normal monthly blood work done throughout the year. Some months my drugs may have been tweaked a little and for a few months, Dr. Cordova discontinued a drug or two.

I did have an appointment in May because of shortness of breath and becoming tired very quickly. It just so happens, Dr. Cordova wanted to talk to me about my blood work that was completed in April.

Epstein Barr Virus (EBV) was detected in my April blood test. Most people are infected by EBV in early childhood. It usually causes no symptoms or only a brief, mild illness.

When teens or young adults become infected, it can cause infectious mononucleosis or "mono." The symptoms of mono are extreme fatigue, fever, sore throat, and swollen lymph nodes. To control this virus, Dr. Cordova stopped some and changed some of the drugs I was currently on and added a few more. The two they stopped were cellcept and prograf and started me on Imuran and cyclosporin respectively.

Next, after two plus years, he thought my heart rate (HR) was low and wanted me to see an electro physiologist to evaluate why it is low. My heart rate runs anywhere from 56 – 64. Dr. Cordova told me this was the heart rate of an athlete, and I didn't quite fit the bill for being an athlete. Here I was building myself up for a compliment, which I didn't get. We'll see how this all works out!

He gave me a script to have an

"02 UPTAKE CARDIOPULMONARY EXERCISE" completed. A cardiopulmonary exercise test (cpet) is the gold standard for evaluating symptom-limiting exercise intolerance in patients with suspected respiratory or cardiac disease. Dr. Cordova wanted to see me again the following month to follow-up on the EBV and the other tests he ordered. He just couldn't do just one test; Dr. Cordova also had to order a ekg and a CT scan. These tests, he allowed me to have done at Penn State Hershey Medical Center (PSHMC). At our following appointment, we looked at each of the tests he wanted and he was satisfied with the results, but he still didn't think I have the body of an athlete.

Anyways, back to reality… my breathing sucks and it is no better than it was in previous months. We revisited the meds, and of course, there had to be a change in some of them and, a tweak to others.

At the end of my September appointment, Dr. Cordova mentioned something to us about the possibility of a re-transplant if it should become necessary sometime in the future. This was something we haven't even thought about, even as a remote possibility.

The best part of the visit is my transplanted lung is clear and strong!

I will end this year on a semi high note… although I had EBV and may still have it, I tire easily, blood levels are not exactly where they should be, sometimes I have a hard time breathing, and I may be looking at a possible second transplant, I am still here and thrilled to be here. I still put my faith and confidence in my team, and GOD, and if they are happy with my recovery and they can control all that is happening to me with medicines and treatments, then I am happy also. Let's get to 2017!

<u>**2017**</u>

A few paragraphs back, I said the EBV was gone. Today, this was a true statement, but I have had flareups of the EBV over the years. Maybe now I might be able to say it is gone, but I will guess at some time in the future I might deal with it again.

The month started off rather hectic for me. Of course, we had our traditional New Year's dinner of pork and sauerkraut and got our fill of college football.

 As part of my required testing, I had a DEXA Scan. This is a test to make certain my bones are not becoming brittle because of all the meds I am taking. The last thing I would need is a broken bone.

I had my follow-up appointment, and Dr. Cordova says the EBV levels on my monthly blood test are rising. This is becoming a pain since the last two months have shown it had disappeared. Another change in my drugs and they will monitor via my monthly blood draws. Other than this, his only comment was for me to continue exercising and stay active.

I don't like to get too excited, but this period of time has been the least active medically since my transplant. Oh sure, I have had my monthly blood draws, flare ups of my EBV and my scheduled appointments, but everything has been pretty good. Nothing too extraordinary, even the changes in meds have decreased. I feel good! I have been blessed and I know it. My next appointment will be next year.

This year has been pretty active for me. Earlier I stated we normally had a Valentine couples' weekend at the beach. This year just the husbands went for a long weekend. You know where the guys do guy things! Spent Memorial Day weekend at the beach with friends and in July we spent two weeks in Hawaii. In August we traveled to the Midwest to visit family and attend my 25th Infantry Division Military Police reunion from Vietnam. We were able to attend a Phillies game and attended our first Pulmonary Fibrosis Foundation Summit in Nashville. We were able to do all this and still keep up with activities of our families and friends. I almost forgot, I even had a radio interview on one of our local stations to tell my story and to help get the word out about pulmonary fibrosis. I feel so fortunate and blessed to be able to do all of this and more.

Santa Claus was extremely good to me this year. One of my goals since transplant was to get back out on the golf course. (Please bear with me and you will see where I am going with this in a page or two.) You see my current clubs were purchased way back when I returned from Vietnam over 50 years ago. Not that it mattered, but I thought new clubs would improve my game. See, I was thinking again… new clubs apparently had no impact on my game after all.

<u>**2018**</u>

My appointment at Temple was scheduled for January 23, but much has happened before then. We had our traditional pork and sauerkraut dinner to bring us luck and good health in 2018.

Here we are in the midst of flu season, I have my shots and I thought I would be able to escape another season without getting sick. Boy, was I wrong on this thought!

Right after New Year, I was never so sick in all my life with all the flu-like symptoms and probably a few more not known to man. I was in bed and didn't want to eat or drink anything; I didn't even want to see or hear anybody's voice. This was the first time we needed to call our team. For two days they tried to treat what was happening with antibiotics and other meds, changing drugs when one didn't work with something else.

I have been in bed being the good patient and telling Karen I was going to be ok because whatever I have is not transplant related. I was supposed to be one of the three Wisemen for the processional at our church service for Epiphany. Let me say now, this Wiseman didn't make it.

Because I wouldn't eat or drink liquids, I ended up in the hospital for four days to be treated for the flu. Karen called my pulmonologist at PSHMC at home and she met me at her office. As soon as she saw me, she said, 'You're staying.' After being admitted to the hospital and as soon as they started the IV to get fluid back in my body, I almost immediately started to feel better.

Of course, since I am a transplant recipient, they did more blood work, ekg and an x-ray to make certain there was nothing else to be concerned about. After having everyone worried about me, I was released from the hospital after a short four-day stay. It took me a few days to recover from this bout with the flu. This experience was only the second time I have ever been admitted to a hospital for any reason and I don't want to do it again. The first time was for my transplant.

The moral of this story is the flu shot may not stop you from getting the flu, but it may soften the blow if you do; and for heaven's sake if you are told to drink lots of liquids, don't argue with the wife. It just might keep you out of the hospital.

As long as we are talking about my health, let's get it out of the way. I had four appointments this year with my team at Temple, and for the most part, nothing they were going to say would be unexpected.

After my stay at the Hershey Medical Center, Dr. Cordova wanted to review the tests that were done at Hershey. I did the proverbial pft's and met with Dr. Cordova. He reviewed the results of the tests which were done at PSHMC and was satisfied.

Because of my continued shortness of breath, he did order a VQ scan to examine the air flow and blood flow in my lungs and said we would review the results at our next appointment. VQ is really two scans in one. The first test looks to see how well the blood flows through my lungs, and the second looks at where the blood flows in my lung. At my next scheduled appointment, we did review the results and all seemed to be in order.

He looked at the CT scan and noted the right lung or native lung is more fibrotic and decreasing in size. Decreasing in size is normal. It's normal since that lung is not being used very much.

Dr Cordova noted my FVC and FEV1 continue to slip and are probably contributing to my tiring and shortness of breath.

Since the pft's I complete at each visit continue to drop, he once again mentioned I might be looking at another transplant. This time they would replace the right lung. I really believe he is just preparing me for what is to come.

After watching my blood pressure for a few months, Dr. Cordova decided my blood pressure is way too high and I should get my blood pressure under control. Of course, this meant taking another pill or two. Coreg (carvedilol) is the pill of choice for my blood pressure. "I just don't seem to be able to catch a break of late!"

This year Karen and I were selected to be Ambassadors for the Pulmonary Fibrosis Foundation (PFF). The PFF Ambassador Program encourages patients and caregivers to become spokespeople for the Pulmonary Fibrosis community on behalf of the Pulmonary Fibrosis Foundation. (Say this sentence quick three times). Ambassadors offer hope and inspiration to others affected with Pulmonary Fibrosis by speaking about their experiences and promoting disease awareness on behalf of the PFF.

Karen and I jumped at the opportunity to become Ambassadors to tell our story as a twosome who have been on the same journey with a fatal disease which has no known cause, no known effective treatment and no known cure. The only difference is one of us, me, is the patient and the other, her, is the caregiver.

I believe the PFF agrees our stories are worth telling. Karen has been on this same journey with me from the very beginning. She has not missed any of my doctor appointments or tests I have had since 2009 when I started on this journey.

Since we have been on this journey together from the start, why wouldn't we want to continue together? After all, we are *Partners for Life* aren't we? If you are wondering, I borrowed this part from a friend of mine, Jim Uhrig, who wrote a book about his journey with Pulmonary Fibrosis.

As PFF Ambassadors, Karen and I have had the opportunity to travel across this United States sharing our story about this dreaded disease. We have met with support groups in not only PA but IL, NM, AZ, NY, and one of us, not me, had the opportunity to travel to HI for a support group meeting.

I keep preaching about staying active and not sitting around the house and doing nothing. This goes for those who are pre- transplant as well as post-transplant patients. You have to remain as healthy as possible.

During this time, we kept up with our volunteer commitments. Some of our commitments include meals-on-wheels food deliveries, speaking engagements for the PFF and Donate Life, continuing with pulmonary rehab, volunteering at a local homeless mission, attending a grandson's high school graduation. We also had time with our families and friends which is very important to us. I have mentioned several times before about giving back to the pulmonary fibrosis community. Since my transplant, we have volunteered our time to many local organizations to get the word out about this disease and share our story about our journey with IPF.

One thing out of the ordinary we did was host a casual picnic for members of our support group who have had a lung transplant at Temple. There are eleven of us who have connections to the transplant team there. Eight attended and we spent much time-sharing stories and comparing notes about our journeys. Sadly, one of those in attendance has passed away and is now breathing easy.

We try to pay back to the pulmonary fibrosis community and September22nd being my 5th "lungaversary," we had the opportunity to prepare a dinner meal for the guests staying at the Gift of Life Family House in Philadelphia. This is something enjoyed by all.

I have made it to the five-year post-transplant mark. Many post lung transplant recipients, on average, are given three to five years to survive this disease that none of us asked for. Remember this three to five years number that has been crammed down our throats… it's just that… a number.

Here we are at the end of 2018 and looking forward to what 2019 might have in store for me.

<u>**SECTION II:**</u>

<u>**2019 – Infinity**</u>!

<u>**2019**</u>

Happy New Year Everyone! I had my pork and sauerkraut today and now I should have good luck for the rest of the year.

Okay, I think I did a pretty good job of keeping SECTION ONE pretty brief considering it covered four-years of my journey.

Please don't think everything was hunky-dory for me, because it wasn't. As you saw, I did have a few issues, most of which have been corrected, but I still carry some of them into this section. I must admit, more detail is provided in what follows.

So, let's get started with the next part of my journey…

<u>**January – March 2019**</u>

If I could just get rid of feeling tired and short of breath, I think I would be a little happier. Other than blood tests, seeing my PCP and having a Dexa-Scan (Bone Density), I have no other appointments at Temple until mid-March

Other than the above-mentioned tests/appointments, the rest of the time was mainly devoted to our volunteer commitments, support groups, catching up with friends and family and a long weekend at the beach. Even in February the salt air smells great.

This month started with a visit to the local Veteran Administration (VA) clinic for my annual checkup. Even though I had my first transplant at Temple University Hospital in Philadelphia, being a Veteran, I get some of my medications from the VA. In order to get those prescribed medications, I must see a VA doctor and have a physical at least once a year. I do this because some of the transplant drugs are quite expensive, and at the VA, most of them cost me 24 dollars for a 90-day supply. If you are a Veteran, be sure you check out what VA benefits you might be eligible for. The outcome of this visit was more a social visit than anything, and Dr. Cho found me healthy, considering the circumstances.

My next stop was to see my cardiologist for a check-up and as expected, the heart is still strong, and no problems were detected, and I get to go back in another six months.

Here we are, three months after my last visit to Temple. All the tests ordered in December were reviewed, and Dr. Cordova seemed happy with the results.

I was still dealing with the shortness of breath and tiring so quickly. He changed my meds again, and again was hinting at another transplant sometime down the road, maybe sooner rather than later.

Karen and I will be going on a Rhine River cruise in Europe, and we wanted to make sure we had the blessing of the team to go. We got the approval of the team and Dr. Cordova. He prescribed an antibiotic (levofloxacin) to take along with me in the unlikely event I would get sick. My next visit would be in July after we return from vacation.

My next stop was the dentist office for my six months check-up. I got a good report, no cavities, and I get to go back in six months. Remember, keeping your teeth and mouth in good shape is part of the pre-transplant evaluation routine. They want to eliminate any cause of infection you might be exposed to.

Other than the above-mentioned tests/appointments, the rest of the time was mainly devoted to our volunteer commitments, support groups, catching up with friends and family and, add to the list, following our grandkids sports activities.

April – June

This three-month period was basically doctor visit free. Don't get me wrong-I did have my periodic blood tests, which have become part of my normal routine.

Well, we were able to check another box off our bucket list. We took that Rhine River cruise. We decided against an ocean cruise, too many people on a cruise ship; we thought about a cruise on one of the rivers here in the states which piqued our interest until we heard about this one. When we get to take another cruise, we will do one of the rivers in the United States.

We flew into Zurich, Switzerland, and stayed there for two nights before taking a bus to Basil and got on our boat for an eight-day cruise. We saw many beautiful sights and tasted some great local wines and beer along the way. The boat stopped at cities in Switzerland, France, Germany, and Holland.

Other than vacation, the rest of our time was mainly devoted to our volunteer commitments, support groups, catching up with friends, participating in health fairs, and doing presentations for Donate Life, family, and, add to the list, following our grandkids sports activities. It seems we are more active now than we ever were.

July

This month started out sort of like the previous few months have… slow, no doctors' appointments until near the end of the month, so it was just us doing our normal things: golf, volunteer commitments, family and friends… well you get the picture, but things were soon to change and not necessarily for the better!

The second Tuesday of July while on the golf course, I just couldn't finish the round I was playing, and, if you know me, if I paid to play 18 holes, I wanted to get my money's worth. But this week, playing the entire 18 holes was out of the question; it just wasn't going to happen. I became so tired and short of breath I just couldn't continue. I hate to admit it, but I surrendered to the course and struggled home.

Let me explain how this whole thing started… golf was going pretty well through June, and then I needed to stop because of our planned vacation. When we returned from vacation, I started playing again, but something was just not right with me. I was getting extremely short of breath and still tiring quite quickly, more so than previously. Now seven years ago, I could probably blame it on my age and not being in better physical shape, but this wasn't what I was feeling. We all know when something is not the way it should be with our bodies.

Just a side note, if you were paying attention, two pages ago I may have suggested I tasted some of the European wines and beers on our travels. To put my mind at ease and yours too, Dr. Cordova says this had nothing to do with this relapse.

To make a long golfing story short, this July day was the last day I played golf in 2019.

<u>August</u>

I had to make an appointment to see Dr. Cordova, and we were off to Temple to try and find out what is going on with me. As always, a trip to the pft lab was in order before I saw Dr. Cordova. I also needed to have a CT scan and an x-ray which were completed earlier in the day.

My bloodwork was normal, CT scan showed nothing out of the ordinary and the x-rays were negative. However, my pft's showed a big decline in my FVC and FEV1 and because of my extreme shortness of breath, Dr. Cordova suspected I was starting to go through chronic rejection. To be certain of his diagnosis, he scheduled a bronchoscopy to be sure. A bronchoscopy is an endoscopic medical procedure used to look inside the airways (bronchi) and the lungs. It involves inserting a bronchoscope—a narrow tube which has a light and a camera on one end—through the nose or mouth and guiding it down through the trachea (windpipe) in order to get an internal view of the respiratory system. The test results came back with finding nothing to be concerned about.

In order to be proactive with treatment, they increased my prednisone to 10mg, increased my azithromycin to 100mg, put me on an Advair inhaler and ordered more blood work before I return for my next appointment.

This possible chronic rejection was not something we were prepared to hear about after almost six years of almost normal living. Don't get me wrong, I did encounter a few bumps in the road since my transplant, but they were minor compared to what we thought might be happening now. The goal is to stop or slow the progression of the chronic rejection, if that is what I am dealing with.

 I was bummed to hear my body had finally figured out I had a lung which wasn't part of the original equipment package which came with this body of mine, and now it may be trying to reject the lung and me along with it!

I returned for a follow-up appointment in late August and it was confirmed what I was experiencing was chronic rejection. I had hoped Dr. Cordova's suspicions were wrong, but deep down I knew what was happening.

I was diagnosed with "Bronchiolitis Obliterans Syndrome," BOS for short.

What is BOS you are wondering? BOS is scarring of the small airways of my transplanted lung. This scarring leads to the narrowing of the airways, limiting airflow with loss of lung function. Early after the onset of BOS, I may not have had any symptoms, but I developed the breathlessness and cough as BOS. got worse.

The next question you might ask would be how is BOS treated? Good question! Just like anything else associated with the pulmonary fibrosis/idiopathic pulmonary fibrosis we are dealing with, there is no good answer. In my case, the

250mg of azithromycin, an antibiotic I have been taking, has been increased to 500mg and my cellcept, an immuno suppression drug, has been increased to 1000mg twice a day and then all we are hoping for is this may help slow or reverse the decline in my lung function; it won't cure me.

Finally, if the changes made above and BOS continues to progress, and if my lung function continues to decline and if it becomes severe enough, then I may have to be evaluated for another transplant. Note the "ifs" in this sentence, nothing is etched in stone. Through this entire journey of mine I have found this disease has been full of "ifs!"

For those of you reading this who have been diagnosed with IPF, does any of what I have written in the last few paragraphs sound familiar?

Well, how about adding another 3-letter acronym to your vocabulary: Idiopathic Pulmonary Fibrosis *(IPF)*. You probably never heard of until you were diagnosed. Bronchiolitis Obliterans Syndrome (BOS), you might not have heard of until you saw it in the last few paragraphs I have written!

With IPF there is nothing to cure this disease. Even with Ofev and Esbriet you can only slow the progression of IPF, it won't cure it. At the present time we are treating **BOS** by increasing the dosage of some of my drugs and adding others, hoping to slow the progression.

Dr. Cordova did present an option that could possibly help me. He suggested I may be eligible for a study being conducted by Washington University in St. Louis, MO. It is a study using photopheresis to treat lung disease. This is not a new study. It has been used somewhat successfully to treat chronic rejection in heart transplants and some types of cancer, but it has not been approved by the FDA for lung disease. Once again, this treatment is not a cure but rather something to hopefully slow the progression of the scaring in the bronchia. The outcomes could be your breathing remains the same, gets better, or you continue to get worse. Oh, what a choice!

Without going into a lot of detail, to qualify for this study it is based on low FVC & FEV1 numbers. Those numbers would need to be low and continue to show a decline over a period of time to qualify for this study.

If accepted into the study I would be required to enter an aggressive program where I would be subject to the cleansing of my blood. Similar to dialysis, some of my blood would be removed from my body run through a machine, the white blood cells would be separated, cleaned with ultra violet light and then returned to my body.

I was accepted as a candidate for this study. All I had to do was show three consecutive pft's showing a decline in the FEV1 and FVC. It took me to May of 2021 for me to officially start.

Unfortunately for me, this turned out to be a slow process. My numbers fluctuated each time I had a pft. I was considered a "provisional" candidate. In other words, I would be carried on program for six months and then if my numbers were not good, I would be removed from the program.

September

My next appointment was in mid-September and my breathing was not any better. Of course, they had to increase/change some of my meds again. I thought I was at the point where the number of pills I was taking each day was getting less; instead, they have been increasing.

Having my pft numbers drop has not been a sure thing. In fact, the FEV1 increased and no decrease was noted in the FVC. I was sent to the sidelines again. Oh well, I will try again on my next trip to Philly. Temple tried to get a waiver from the sponsor to allow me to participate in the program, but it was denied.

This visit, Dr. Cordova again brought up the subject of possibly another transplant for me sometime in the future. It was a general discussion of what if? Dr. Cordova suggested it is probably too early to start the process, but the idea has firmly been implanted into our minds. He indicated if and when the transplant would occur, I would receive a single right lung. This would be my native lung. I guess in reality the right lung is essentially just there doing next to nothing.

I have said before, we try to pay back to the pulmonary fibrosis community and the 22nd being my 6th "lungaversary" we had the opportunity to prepare a dinner meal for the guests staying at the Gift of Life Family House. This is something enjoyed by all.

October

I don't go to Temple until the 14th so the days up until then had been pretty normal, whatever the word normal means in the world I live in.

Along with our normal activities we are committed to attend a PFF function at National Harbor, near Washington D.C. for their annual walk. This walk raises money for their organization so they can continue to help the PFF community and do research to find a cure for this dreadful disease. I think I must clarify what walking I did… I walked as far as the first park bench and waited for Karen and daughter to return. Keep in mind I still tire and get out of breath quickly so I did have an excuse.

Before my appointment with Dr. Cordova, I had to have my pft's and an x-ray. We reviewed all the testing. He was satisfied with the x-ray, but still was concerned with the pft's. He looked at a previous CT scan and saw what he thought might be a small hiatal hernia and wanted me to see a gastrointestinal (G.I.)) doctor. A gastroenterologist specializes in preventing, diagnosing and treating conditions of the gastrointestinal (GI) tract, or digestive system. This includes the esophagus, stomach, intestines, liver, pancreas and gallbladder. A GI specialist focuses on the health needs of adults with digestive problems.

I just can't catch a break. If it is not one thing it's another!

<u>November</u>

My next appointment was on November 4th, so what do we decide to do… drive out to South Bend, IN to visit our son and attend a Notre Dame football game on November 2. Our daughter and family from West Bend, WI are also coming for the weekend. It was great for all of us to get together, but it was a very cold weekend for a football game for me. Everyone else went to the game, and I stayed at the house and kept warm.

This was not the dumbest thing we did. Keep in mind I have an appointment in Philadelphia on the 4th which is Monday. What do we do? We get up early Sunday morning, we all go to breakfast and then we hit the turnpike and head east to the City of Brotherly Love. We arrived late Sunday evening, and fortunately for us, we had reservations at the Gift of Life Family House and they waited for us. This was a total of almost 700 miles, and it took us about 11 hours to complete the journey. Whoever said 'old people' don't do some stupid things!

Nothing has really changed with my symptoms and how I feel. I still tire quickly and get out of breath quickly, even walking short distances. My pft's show I am not yet ready for the photopheresis study. Dr. Cordova also wants me to do pulmonary rehab and gave me a script for this. He wants to make sure I remain fit and active.

This was also the appointment where Dr. Cordova said it was probably time to get me listed for a second transplant or a "re-transplant" as they call it. If nothing else, I will be on the list; and if anything, drastic happens, I will at least have some of the testing done. I realize some of the testing may need to be repeated. I guess this was sort of a double edge sword… I need to be sick enough to need a transplant and healthy enough to survive the surgery and recovery. I made the decision to move forward with this process. As Larry the Cable guy would say… **GitRdone!**

When this happens, I am certain I will feel a little odd... having two different lungs, from two different donors doing the breathing for me and helping to keep me alive.

I told Dr. Cordova my answer was yes; I would accept a lung if offered.

When I had my first transplant it was more difficult for me, or in this case us, to make the ultimate decision for me to say yes. I went through all of the same emotions many of you may have had to go through when you made your decision. One would think it would be an easy decision to make, but it's not... it really isn't!

December

I did get an appointment with the G.I. doctor at Temple, and it just happens to be the same day as my appointment with my doctor. This appointment showed I had Gerd, another word for acid reflux. In order to fix this, they would need to do a fundoplication procedure. A Nissen fundoplication is a surgery to correct gastroesophageal reflux disease (GERD). The surgery tightens the junction between the esophagus and the stomach to prevent acid reflux. The esophagus is the tube between your mouth and stomach. It is part of your gastrointestinal (GI) system.

Dr. Cordova also ordered a manometry test where they run a tube through your nose into your stomach for 24 hours to see how much reflux I really have.

I did my pft's and they were nothing to brag about, a six-minute walk which I now assume might be used as a base line, changed a couple of meds and was told to return in six weeks. The G.I. doctor prescribed a med for my acid reflux.

It couldn't be Prilosec which I could get over the counter; no it had to be a prescribed version of the same drug.

2019 has not been the greatest of years for me, but it certainly could have been worse.

On the good side, I was able to remain active for the most part, did some traveling, played a few rounds of golf and even had time for family, especially my wife, and friends, and I have the chance to be listed for another transplant. Hopefully I will get into the photopheresis study which may serve as a bridge until I get my transplant.

The real downer is going through chronic rejection and not knowing what my future really holds for me.

Hopefully 2020 will be a better year for all of us!

<u>**2020**</u>

<u>**January – February**</u>

Here we are, leaving 2019 behind us and heading into a bright new year. For me, I think 2020 will be a good year, after all, what else could happen while I am on this journey?

It didn't take long for me to find out what lay ahead for me. I really thought January and February would fly by without many issues. But you will see, I may be a little off target with this statement. By mid-January I was in the midst of my pre-transplant evaluations. I needed to have many of the same tests I completed eight years earlier.

Some of those tests and meetings were with doctors, nurses, surgeons, psychologists, nutritionists, cardiologists, speech pathologists, and social workers. Also, during this period, I was poked, prodded, and jabbed in various ways and places. I had tests coming out the ole wazoo! I had CT scans, chest x-rays, EKGs, echocardiograms, a tine test to make certain I didn't have TB, pulmonary function tests, six-minute walks, a muga scan, a maximum exercise test, psychological testing, lung scan, DEXA scan, Doppler study, heart catherization, barium swallow, and probably a few other tests I can't recall or probably don't want to recall.

All of the tests were performed on various days at Temple University Hospital, my transplant hospital. Some of the days I had several tests and meetings with doctors, and on other days it was just one test or appointment. None of the tests I completed would deter me from my decision to move forward with a possible transplant. I needed to talk to Dr. Shigemura, the transplant surgeon; he wanted to know why I wanted a transplant. My immediate response was I wanted a quality of life and to be able to breathe again without difficulty.

At the time of this interview, I was not on oxygen and have not been since being diagnosed with chronic rejection. Because of not being on oxygen, I was told he could not support me being listed at the present time. I was disappointed by this meeting. Here I am struggling to breath. Because I am not on oxygen and only because I was not on oxygen, I was not being given the opportunity to be listed for transplant at the present time.

The only tests left to be completed were a colonoscopy and a manometry. The Team allowed me to do them closer to home and they would accept the results. All of these test results were accepted and now all they needed to do was present my case to the panel. Things now started to go slower than I would like; Karen kept reminding me I must be patient. Again, this patience thing comes up.

In February I had my first MOHS surgery to remove a basil cell carcinoma which was benign.

MOHS surgery is a painstakingly slow procedure. It requires microscopic analysis of tissue cells while the surgery is taking place. The borders of each thin layer of tissue are analyzed for potential malignancy as they are removed horizontally. This technique is designed to remove the entire tumor with minimal amounts of healthy tissue. This results in less disfigurement. This is something we have to deal with as transplant patients, especially if we spend a lot of time outdoors. We need to use sunscreen when we are outside and cover our bare spots.

I continue to struggle with my chronic rejection, my number one priority at the present time. I must continue to do whatever I need to do to stay as healthy as possible and hope the drugs I am taking slows the progression. I think this is something I can handle for the time being.

March

They say March comes in like a lion and goes out like a lamb. Well, so far this month the lion has come in and is not showing any signs of leaving his den. It wasn't long until we were introduced to a new word. As Big Bird would say…. Can you say… COVID-19?

On March 6, an emergency disaster declaration was announced in response to the presence of the 2019 novel coronavirus (COVID-19) in Pennsylvania. COVID-19 is a severe respiratory disease, resulting in illness or death, caused by person-to-person spread of the virus. Commonly reported symptoms of COVID-19 infection include fever, cough, and shortness of breath.

March 7th, we attended a birthday party for our daughter, and on the 8th, Karen and I decided we were going to start our own "self-imposed quasi-isolation" until we find out more information about this COVID-19 thing.

At first, like most, I didn't think much about the word COVID-19. Like many, this word never really resonated with me until the death toll began to rise. Unfortunately, as I sit here and write in February, the death toll has risen to more than 900,000 people.

I have talked about being and remaining active during our journey with IPF. This is going to slow us down for a while until we get used to what is happening around us and make adjustments to our daily routines. I have shared how active we have been throughout our journey. Now all of a sudden everything that was in person has suddenly changed to Zoom-type meetings or just cancelled altogether. Meals-on-Wheels, Support Groups, Pulmonary Fibrosis meetings, and church all cancelled or done via Zoom or other electronic means.

My journey during this period of COVID-19 has probably been much like yours. I try to stay safe and as healthy as possible. The more I listened to those who were supposedly in the know and those not in the know, the more confused I became. Besides, whatever was suggested today as fact will surely change or be modified in some way tomorrow. I had to decide who or what I was going to believe and for me following the science was my best option. Besides, I have listened to my doctors for 10 plus years and I find no reason not to follow their advice now.

Since COVID began, we really have not been out of our house or had any real contact with people. Now don't get me wrong, we do the necessary things like pick up our groceries we had ordered on line; we go to the drugstore to get my drugs. We haven't really seen our kids, relatives or friends other than to have a short porch visit. We have not been in a restaurant, although we might do takeout once in a while.

Who would have thought we would be wearing a mask if we were to go out in public or to a business and schools, churches or restaurants would be closed and people out of a job?

Zoom becomes a word we became all too familiar with… we attended church, school, visits with family, and even our doctors' appointments were held via zoom.

Personally, of all the Zoom meetings I was fortunate to have, I did not like to talk to my doctors via Zoom or telephone appointments. I felt and still do feel the in-person appointments were and are more beneficial, especially since I was dealing with chronic rejection during this period, I knew other tests and procedures could be needed. However, I do understand the safety implications.

To summarize what has happened during this three-month period: I completed my transplant evaluation program and was not listed because of not being on oxygen; COVID-19 decides to raise havoc with the world; and I am still dealing with chronic rejection. This about sums things up in a nutshell!

<u>April</u>

Since COVID-19 kicked in, one would assume writing would be easier, but it really isn't. Yes, a lot of the fun things we did came to a screeching halt. No more outdoor activities, going to the beach or even following the activities of our grandchildren. Whatever visiting was to be done was done from a social distance, wearing a mask or using the new word we learned… Zoom. Support group meetings and webinars all done electronically. A day out for us consisted of picking up our groceries we had ordered on-line and maybe go for a short car ride.

I was supposed to go to Temple for an in-person appointment with my doctor, do a six-minute walk and pft's.

This appointment was moved to a telephone interview. This was my first, and I hoped my last appointment which is not in person. To me it was sort of awkward being able to talk to Dr. Cordova but not able to see him. I take my vitals every day and log them just in case I ever needed them for a telephone appointment. (Just in case you didn't get it, I was being a little sarcastic there.) He still wants to keep me stable and in the best of health he can so there was no change in meds.

The bombshell of this visit was this: he talked to the transplant surgeon and asked him to reconsider my case and asked to be able to present me to the team which selects the transplant candidates. After consideration, he allowed me to proceed with the transplant process. Finally, now I thought things would start to move a little faster.

May

On May 10th I was officially listed for a "re-transplant." I questioned why it was called "re-transplant" since it was my native right lung which was the one being transplanted. I was told since I already had one transplant, anything after that would be considered a re-transplant. I thought this day would never come, but it did, and I was finally listed. My LAS was still low, at 34, the same as it was for my 1st transplant back in 2013. Last time my wait was only a little more than three months. This would be wishful thinking on my part if it happened this way again.

Now, the wait begins and all of the preparation for my second transplant starts. Well, the wait begins for all of us, but Karen is the one needing to have a suitcase packed and ready to go at a moment's notice. I must admit she is well prepared for when the call comes. She has a list of things she needs to gather from each room in our house to take with her for her part of this journey. Everything I would initially need could be put in a brown paper bag because I would be provided with what seemed like an endless supply of hospital gowns. I must admit, I did pack a backpack to take with me this time

Since the very beginning, I have been saying how important it is to remain active and not become sedentary. I know COVID-19 has affected all of us, our activities are limited, but we certainly have the ability to walk around our neighborhoods or properties for some exercise. If worse would come to worse, we can even walk around the interior of our homes.

June – August

June definitely was an uneventful month; no outside activities other than zoom meetings that have been arranged. We didn't even have a July 4th cookout.

July was much the same, only I did meet with my team. I was supposed to see them at Temple, but my in-person visit was changed to a phone appointment.

Doctor Cordova wanted me to start pulmonary rehab again and I agreed the exercise would be a good idea. Now because of the COVID shut downs, I asked where he would suggest I do pulmonary rehab. He also wants me to get into the photopheresis program as soon as my pft's cooperate. If my pft's go down, he will see me in two weeks; otherwise, it will be three months until my next appointment.

<u>**September**</u>

Well, you can copy what I said for my August activities to the month of September. Zoom and phone call meetings are starting to be a pain. I hope this COVID thing soon starts to go away and we return to normal, whatever normal might be. My pft's must not have dropped too drastically since I had no two-week appointment. But rather he stretched it out to four weeks.

I have had a few tele-appointments, and quite frankly, I don't like them. I understand why they are necessary, but I still find them so impersonal. I requested my next appointment be in person. I will see how I make out on this request. Bottom line is I am stable. I guess this is good in the grand scheme of things.

I may not have been able to see my own doctor in person, but somehow, I was able to see an ear, nose and throat specialist in person at Temple. This doesn't make sense to me… oh well, I don't make the rules. Anyways, when this doctor walked into the exam room, I immediately thought I was going to be quarantined for some unknown reason. He was covered head to toe in protective gear and I mean head to toe in protective gear! Oh well I got a chuckle out of this until he ran a little scope down my throat to see into my stomach to check for acid reflux (Gerd). They have been talking about doing a fundoplication for quite some time, and I think they are just now getting all their ducks in a row. I know this procedure can be done either pre- or post-transplant. In my simple medical mind, it would make sense to do this procedure pre-transplant when the patient is probably stronger, but what do I know.

Well, it has been four months, since I was listed. This was about the amount of time I waited for my first transplant after being listed. In the perfect world I think I live in, I should have received the call for my second transplant. I know, I know this was wishful thinking on my part. I am quite aware of the fact there are people sicker and my time will come when the man upstairs says it is time.

I had one telephone appointment at Temple. The Ear Nose & Throat doctor called to follow up on the manometry procedure he did earlier. I told him all was well and I could tell no difference. He called in a prescription for a higher dosage of Prilosec which I could not get over the counter. All this for someone who wasn't aware he had acid reflux and to this day still doesn't.

The most exciting thing that has happened to me this month is my seven-year anniversary of my first transplant. I continue to outlive the statistics for those who have had a single lung transplant.

Another month in the books. Not much has really changed since last month as far as activities are concerned. We continue to do Zoom meetings for support groups with the PFF, Donate Life and several other groups.

If I could breathe without tiring like I did several years ago, I would say I am good or at least better, but things still seem to be going downhill quicker than I would like. Even though I continue to say things suck as far as my health is concerned, I continue to hang strong.

October

My first stop this month is to see my cardiologist at PSHMC. I haven't had an appointment with him since last year, so this is just a routine follow-up visit. Using test results provided by Temple, he concluded with all of their findings. He encouraged a change in diet to include fruits and vegetables and said he will see me next year unless something drastic changes. I will take this as a sign of good visit.

November

I guess I was just lucky or maybe the squeaky wheel does get the attention, but I did get an in-person appointment at Temple at the beginning of this month.

This was day 275 of our self-imposed quasi-isolation we were in. This had nothing to do with this appointment, but I just wanted to throw this little tidbit of worthless knowledge out there!

We talked about my continued shortness of breath, especially when doing steps and inclines. We talked about the potential COVID-19 vaccine which is supposedly on the horizon. He told me Temple was still undecided at this point and for me to wait until I heard from them. He still wants to see me admitted to the photopheresis program if possible.

Dr. Cordova called me the following morning and talked about the fundoplication process. He decided to do it now rather than wait until after the transplant. Remember, back in September I said they were prepping me for a fundoplication; well, it's time. He said someone from thoracic surgery would call me. He also noted while reviewing x-rays and CT scans he saw what he thought might be a cyst on my kidney and wanted me to have it checked out. Here we go, now I get to see another surgeon and a nephrologist. It just never ends!

Unless something drastic happens, I do not have to return until sometime in January.

December

December definitely was an uneventful month, no outside activities other than zoom meetings have been arranged. Didn't even have a big Christmas dinner at Temple this year. I suppose maybe everyone was a little lower key this time of the year and wanted to make certain we patients had a Merry Christmas! Nah, that couldn't be it, after all we are dealing with the medical profession and I am finding out they are good at dropping surprises on us no matter the time of year. Merry Christmas everyone.

I will admit some positives came out of COVID-19. I learned to play many different types of games during our quasi-self-imposed isolation. I read more books than I thought I would. Karen is a puzzler, I bet she completed 30 plus puzzles. Me, on the other hand, I don't have the patience to look for those little pieces of puzzle and put them together. We both agreed we even talked more and talking is always a good thing. Other than the isolation, the COVID-19 and not being around others, the quarantine hadn't been bad.

Talk about being hit with a triple whammy, how about having to deal with COVID-19, chronic rejection all while waiting for another single lung transplant!

As I sit here and write, it has been over a year since I have been diagnosed with chronic rejection; 256 days since Karen and I have started our quasi-self-imposed quarantine; and seven months since I have been listed for a second transplant. I, like many of you, had much on our plate to deal with in 2021, and we have much to be thankful for. Let's hope this new year will be all each of us hope for. Happy New Year!

We did it, or we survived it, or at least we endured it, or whatever the appropriate words are, 2020 is behind us!

Who would have thought we would still be dealing with this COVID-19 pandemic for almost a year? For Karen and I, we will start our second year of our quasi-self-imposed isolation on March 14th.

Oh, don't get me wrong. We haven't turned in to recluses or anything, but we have been very careful as to whom we are exposed or where we go.

The last time we were truly out among people was March 7th of last year when we attended a birthday party. We have not eaten in a restaurant, shopped at a grocery store, or done any shopping at any store since the beginning of March 2020.

In fact, we do most of our shopping on line. Amazon has become a friend of ours. We do our grocery shopping on line and then go to the store for curbside pick-up. Even our pharmacy would mail my prescription refills to the house.

January

January started slow with blood work, a couple of Zoom support group meetings, a video appointment with the VA and a telephone appointment with Dr. Cordova on the 11th. The VA appointment was cordial and to the point. Looked at my vitals, asked how I was feeling, do I need any refills and I will see you next year.

Dr. Cordova was a little more thorough. Here we looked at the pft's I provided him from PSHMC, and he said my FVC and FEV1 numbers are going down, which is not a good thing for me, but good for getting me closer to getting into the Photopheresis study. Okay, we will try again next month. He wanted me to schedule another 6-minute walk test and have pft's done again at PSHMC before our next visit. He also changed some of my meds again.

We talked about the available COVID-19 vaccines, and he said Moderna or Pfizer would be acceptable. A vaccine had been developed and resistance to getting it to possibly save your life or someone else's life has been reported by some individuals.

My next appointment should be in about two months.

We had been talking about curtailing our Meals on Wheels activities after this coming Friday, the 15th, only because we are doing all we can to avoid COVID-19. Well, our deliveries went without a hitch. We made our 12 stops and went home. Shortly after getting home, we received a call from our church facilitator telling us the Supervisor from Meals on Wheels, who was at the distribution center, had received a phone call from his doctor telling him a COVID test he had taken earlier in the week came back positive.

Our contact with this gentleman was minimal at best, but we still had to quarantine and be tested because of his lack of responsibility to self-quarantine himself after being tested for COVID-19.

Nonetheless, off we went to a local drug store and got tested. We had a few anxious days until we got our results back. Fortunately, both of our tests were negative.

We do not know how many people he came in contact with on Friday morning, but one person was one too many.

We have taken every precaution since March 2020, per the CDC guidelines, and then to have this happen due to one person's negligence is worrisome.

Fortunately, for us, the rest of the month was much less stressful. Most everything else we had scheduled was virtual.

We did need to pick up the groceries we ordered. On January 20, I received my first COVID vaccine shot at our local VA Hospital. Hopefully, for all of our sakes, this vaccine will work. If you haven't received your vaccine yet, it's not too late to get it!

February - April

This month was relatively uneventful. Other than staying as safe as we can, attending Zoom meetings, going outside to pick-up our groceries and me getting my second COVID-19 booster shot on February 13th, all was good. I hope you also received your booster shot.

I had in-person appointments at Temple. I needed to have some of my tests re-done and meet with the transplant surgeon. I had to have an ekg, MRI, PFT, six-minute walk and have a ABG (arterial blood gas) test done. This was an annual visit to keep me on the active transplant list. I also met with my doctor.

Dr. Cordova changed a couple of my medications. My pft's slid a little further, not exactly a good thing for my health, but as stated before, it gets me a little closer to the photopheresis study. One more decline and I am in. Talk about a double-edged sword!

Dr. Cordova now wants to do the fundoplication pre-transplant and will get me an appointment with the appropriate surgeon. I guess the hiatal hernia may have gotten a little bigger.

The rest of the month, except for an appointment with the surgeon who would be doing the laparoscopy surgery, was just like past months have been, more Zoom meetings and little face-to-face contact with anyone.

Our meeting with the thoracic surgeon was thorough. We went over my medical history again: he explained why and how they were going to do the procedure; he explained the risks, saying there could be a 'small' risk' of affecting new transplant if done post. If this would be done pre-transplant, I would be 'inactive' on the list for up to four weeks. The appointment ended with the surgeon saying he would get back to us in a few days. I didn't hear back from anyone, so I made the follow-up call. I found out the surgery had been postponed to sometime in the future. It would have been nice if someone would have had the courtesy to call me and tell me of this decision. Still not really sure what this decision means.

We had the normal plethora of our Zoom meetings and very little of face-to-face contact with friends or family. I, along with many of you, am tired of what we are going through and are very eager to get back to some sort of normality.

I did have another PFT, and my numbers dropped again. This makes three tests in a row and should get me in the photopheresis study. I'll let you know!

May

I did it, I was accepted into the Photopheresis Study. To refresh your memory, I would be required to enter an aggressive program where I would be subject to the cleansing of my blood. Similar to dialysis, a portion of my blood would be removed from my body, run through a machine, the white blood cells would be separated, cleaned with ultra violet light and then returned to my body. Anyways, this is a good thing for me. At least I have something which may slow or halt my chronic rejection.

We met with the people responsible for the study, and they went over all of the details from start to finish.

First off, I had to have a special port, which can only be used for this procedure, surgically inserted into my chest. After the port was inserted, I had to wait one week before my first session. My first session was May 19th. My 25th and final session was to be completed around the first week in November and then the port will be removed.

June

For the next few months my Wednesdays and Thursdays will be tied up with the photopheresis study, and the rest of my world will revolve around those days.

I did meet with Dr. Cordova, and, of course, we went over the medicines I was taking and made adjustments as necessary. My labs were ok, but not great, and this was the reason for the medicine changes.

On Friday the 11th, after spending the previous three days at Temple for my appointments with my doctor and photopheresis, I got a phone call from the Lung Center. It was about 7:15am and the Coordinator at Temple said the surgeon wanted me to be prepared for a transplant. At the present time, I was not the primary recipient, but rather I would be the back-up. It was our understanding the primary may not be a good match and they wanted me to be prepared. I was told until the lung was checked we would not know for certain until later, possibly as late as 4pm. Needless to say, the wait really was a test of my patience.

Well, this ended up as, I guess you could call it, a "dry run," even though we never went to the hospital. It was a good test to see how well we were prepared. Even though it didn't take long for me to put those few items I would need in my backpack I keep at the ready, it took Karen a little longer since she would be staying at the Gift of Life Family House. All in all, it was a good exercise to see how prepared we are. This was the first call I have received about a transplant since I was listed back on May 10, 2020. At least I know they did not lose my phone number.

July

I met with Dr. Cordova and went over my drugs and made necessary adjustments and talked about the slight upswing of my pft's. He told me even though my pft's went up slightly, it was probably too early to determine if it was result of the photopheresis.

Everything else was status quo, and he said I was still stable. So, this is all good. I was to return in two months.

<u>**August**</u>

This month started like any other month we have endured since the pandemic started way back in March of 2020, but it certainly didn't end like any of those.

To refresh your memory, I was listed for another single lung transplant back in May of 2020 and have been waiting anxiously since then for "the call." I know I had a "dry run" back in June, but this is not the same. The call I had been waiting for has been eluding me for almost 465 days since I was listed.

The phone rang around 6:30pm on Monday evening August 9th.. I looked at the phone and it said "Private Caller." Under normal circumstances I would not answer a call I couldn't identify and let a call like this go to voicemail. But there was something different about this call, something different to this day I can't really put my finger on. I answered and it was Ryan from the Transplant Center telling me they had a right lung for me and if I accepted, I needed to come to Temple as soon and as safely as we could get there. I accepted the offer without hesitation and after getting updated about what I needed to do when I arrived at Temple, I said we would be on our way. We finished getting my backpack and Karen's suitcase packed and were ready to hit the PA Turnpike heading east to Temple University Hospital in Philadelphia.

The same emotions which hit me back in 2013 were going through my mind again. The excitement of knowing what we have been waiting for could be close at hand; apprehension, knowing what I am about to go through, there was no guarantee whatsoever the transplant was going to be successful; even a twinge of sadness and guilt knowing while we were pretty excited, we also knew another family was grieving at this very same time.

Karen and I had our moment together, just as we did back in 2013; we held each other, tried to reassure each other everything was going to be alright, shed a tear or two, and I am sure we each said a prayer.

I needed to make five important phone calls to our four kids and my sister telling them what was happening; we were on our way to Temple; the surgery probably would not be until sometime Tuesday morning; I tried to convince everyone that everything was going to be ok. Between the five of them and Karen, everyone who needed to be notified at this time is notified.

We arrived at the hospital shortly before nine and went directly to the Admissions Office where someone was waiting for me. I signed papers, probably most of them were to make certain they were paid for services that were going to be rendered.

We went to the sixth floor to prepare for my surgery the following morning; we were told the transplant surgery would begin somewhere between 5am and 7am. While on this floor I also had an ekg, blood work, chest x-ray, CT scan and they attached the first of many IV's.

They put us in a room and suggested we might want to get some rest. I guess I may have been lucky since they gave me a bed because Karen had to sleep on one of those uncomfortable hospital "visitors chair." I thought I slept soundly, but Karen says we were both restless, I found out later Karen had a concern or two something could go wrong, but she turned her concerns over to GOD, because HE knows what is happening. Don't get me wrong, I also had my concerns, but I was at peace. I put this part of my journey into the hands of GOD and the skillful and steady hands of Dr. Shigemura.

Simplistically this is what I was about to go through: When you're notified that a donor lung is available, you'll be instructed to come to the transplant facility immediately.

When you and your donor lung arrive at the hospital, you'll be prepared for surgery. This includes changing into a colorful hospital gown, receiving an IV, and undergoing general anesthesia. This will put you into an induced sleep. You'll awaken in a recovery room after your new lung is in place.

Your surgical team will insert a tube into your windpipe to help you breathe. Another tube may be inserted into your nose. It will drain your stomach contents. A catheter will be used to keep your bladder empty.

Your surgeon will make a large incision in your chest. Through this incision, your old lung will be removed. Once the new organ is in place, your surgeon connects the pulmonary artery, pulmonary vein and the main airway (bronchus) of the donor organ to the patient's vessels and airway. Drainage tubes are inserted to drain air, fluid, and blood out of the chest for several days to allow the lungs to fully re-expand.

When the new lung is working properly, the incision will be closed. You'll be moved to an intensive care unit (ICU) to recover.

A typical single-lung procedure can take between 4 and 8 hours. A double-lung transfer can take up to 12 hours.

You can expect to remain in the ICU for a few days after the procedure. Your vital signs will need to be closely monitored. Tubes will also be connected to your chest to drain any fluid buildup.

Your entire stay at the hospital could last weeks, but it may be shorter. How long you stay will depend on how well you recover.

Like I said, what I presented is a very simplistic view of a lung transplant and what you might expect.

August 10th

The transplant team came for me at 6:05am and took me to the operating room area. They were still waiting for the final word the lung was good. At 6:35 they got the word and then my journey really begins- I'm off to the operating room (OR)!

Around 1pm I was moved to the Intensive Care Unit (ICU) and Karen finally found out the surgery went well. Karen was a little miffed no one had given her any updates, even when she had asked the nurse on the floor twice to see if she could get any information as to how my surgery was going. It all turned out ok, but I understand her concern.

After getting her official Temple visitor tag, Karen would be allowed into the hospital to visit me. When she came to the ICU, she still had to wait to see me because the doctors were still working their magic on me.

Dr. C talked to her and I believe lessened some of her concerns. He told her all went well with the surgery, answered some of her questions, and told her they did not need to move the heart as much as expected.

Oh, did I forget to mention the heart thing? If you remember, eight years ago, I had a single left lung (SLL) transplant. Eight years is a long time and as my native right lung began to shrink because it wasn't being used as much, my heart started to move into the vacated space around the right lung. It was decided, when I had my transplant, the heart would be moved to where it belonged. Hey, no one said there wouldn't be some little quirky things along the way.

When Karen entered the ICU, the first thing she noticed were the wires! Lots and lots of wires, and like the first time, my arms were strapped so I couldn't move and wouldn't do any harm to myself or rip any of the various tubes or wires out of my body.

I was told I had trouble waking up in the ICU. Karen was with me until 3pm and even though she tried her best to wake me, it was a lost cause.

<u>**August 11th**</u>

I was told Karen arrived around 10am and she told me I was pretty much in the same condition I was in when she left the previous day. She said I was nonresponsive, agitated and thrashing around in bed. For some reason I was taking my time waking up.

They did an in-room bronchoscopy to make certain the lungs were in good shape, no fluid in the lungs and no leaks from all the suturing they did. According to the reports, all was ok. Karen watched the procedure to make certain Dr. Criner was doing it correctly. Since I wasn't responding too well, they inserted a small feeding tube to make certain I had nourishment during my stay in the ICU. A Doppler scan was also ordered to check for possible blood clots, no blood clots were found.

Karen is a real trooper; she stayed with me for most of the day. Although I was not responsive, she kept talking to me and letting me know she was there, but she got no response from me.

<u>**August 12th-**</u>

When Karen got here today, I was awake and talking to anyone who would listen. I figured it was time to wake-up and stop worrying people. They removed my breathing tube and I was breathing on my own. After the breathing tube came out, they had to do another x-ray to make certain the feeding tube was in its appropriate place. It wasn't! They had to re-position the feeding tube and do another x-ray to make certain it was where it belonged. I was told I slept a lot but was coherent.

Dr. Shigemura stopped by to check on me and talked to Karen about my progress. Dr. Cordova was on vacation, but Dr. Shigemura said he was keeping him in the loop about my recovery.

Here is where I need to come clean. The last few days have been quite the blur. In fact, from the time, they put me under to start the operation on August 10th, and until I woke up in the ICU on the 13th, I remember absolutely nothing. What I have written was not necessarily what I remember. Anyways, I want to thank Karen for the great notes she has taken and allowing me to use them to continue my writing. From this point on my memory is not quite as foggy as it has been. Thanks Karen, I love you!

August 13th

I am still in ICU until they find a room for me on the 8th floor in what they call the step-down unit. Today was a good day, I was out of bed for three hours. This was the first time I have been out of bed since before my transplant.

I've found even in the ICU the day starts early. Maybe I should say the ICU is like NYC (New York City) … it never sleeps. All through the night someone is coming into your room checking your vitals or it's time for your medicine.

I suppose the 6am wakeup is more for the convenience of the night shift nurses, so they can get all the patients charts ready to hand over to the day shift. Right after wake up, they are in to do a breathing test, vitals, help getting cleaned up, x-rays and out of bed to wait for the doctors to make their rounds and then time for breakfast.

They turned my oxygen down to 2 LPM (Liters Per Minute), removed my feeding tube and had a Barium Swallow Test today. A barium swallow test is a radiologic examination of the swallowing function using a special movie-type X-ray called fluoroscopy. The patient is observed swallowing various types of substances that can be seen by fluoroscopy (usually liquid barium and/or foods coated with barium) in order to evaluate his or her ability to swallow safely and effectively. They need to make certain food is going into the stomach instead of the lungs. This exam is often performed with a speech/language pathologist present. Unlike my first transplant where it took me almost two months to pass this test, this time I passed it on the first try.

August 14

Another day starts early, same routine as the previous days. A very restless and sleepless night, a lot of activity on the floor. Anyways, I am up, had my face washed, ate my breakfast and sitting in a chair ready for whatever this day brings.

I was taken off oxygen today and now I am breathing only room air. I was allowed to brush my teeth for the first time since I was admitted on the August 9th. Boy, did that feel good! One of the nurses must have really liked me… she washed my hair, shaved and even trimmed my beard and moustache. I almost felt normal after this pampering, but I realize I have a way to go. PT (physical therapy) came and took me for a walk around the floor. This was the first time I was out of bed, other than sitting in a chair, since my transplant. I was so weak and my legs were even weaker. I didn't get far on this walk with them. I was surprised at how my body deconditioned in such a short amount of time.

The doctors removed another drain tube today and also a tube they had inserted in my jugular vein. Now I have one drain tube left for them to take out. They also removed the catheter. Now I get to use a bedpan for the duration of my stay here at Temple.

It's moving day... finally a bed/room opened up in the stepdown unit. The stepdown unit is where you go to complete your hospital stay. Here you will do PT to help get your body back in shape. By no means will I be in shape by the time I am discharged, but it is a start. You will also do OT (occupational therapy) to help you get back to somewhat of a normal physical routine.

The move went smoothly enough. I did note I had a room with a view... from my bed I can watch the heli-pad and see any helicopters that landed here at Temple. All of today's activities tired me out and I was eager to get a good night sleep.

Just a note to those of you who are waiting for the call... if you think there is such a thing as a good night's sleep in the hospital, you may want to rethink that idea, because it probably is not going to happen!

August 15

Early to bed, early to rise makes a man have a long day in Temple's Step-Down Unit. Going to sleep does not seem to be a problem-staying asleep is the problem. I guess I can blame it on the surroundings or a bed I'm not used to, but I am having problems sleeping at nights here at the hospital. This will be worth talking to the doctor about when he makes his rounds.

With help I was able to get out of bed to use the bedside commode or to use the bathroom with help, which is my preference, but not necessarily the preferences of my nurses. Hey, they are the ones who had me all twisted up in lines and tubes and don't want me to trip and fall when I get out of bed. If I fall, this would require too much paperwork for the nurses to complete. I keep ringing the bell, and they keep coming to help me.

Same routine in the mornings, not as much activity on the weekends, things slow down and sometimes seem to go into slow motion. Bloodwork still not where they want it, blood pressure still high and getting meds for this, and PT did not come around today.

August 16

Still did not have a good night sleep. The doctor said it could be a couple of things. He mentioned stress from the surgery, unfamiliar surroundings, noise, etc.… he said he would see if some medication tonight would help me sleep.

Today was a slow day. I was up early and, in my chair, even before the nurses made their first rounds of the new shift. X-rays, blood draw, breathing test, PT, Social Worker and the nurses taking everyone's vitals for the umpteenth time so far today. All in all, I felt pretty good today.

Karen went back home today for a short respite and to recharge her batteries. The Care Partner in our **journey plays an important role in our recovery. They need to be able to have time** to themselves also. She will be back tomorrow and will be here at the hospital to visit with me until they discharge me.

<u>**August 17**</u>

Today was an extremely long day for me. I know what you must be thinking-today is just as long as any other day and this day also has 24 hours in it. That's true, but today I had no visitors. This seemed odd, but I fully understand the reasoning. Because of COVID-19 the hospital was limiting the number of visitors each patient could see. During this period of time, their protocol was to allow one visitor per patient per day, and since my daily visitor was back in Harrisburg, that is the reason my day was so long.

<u>**August 18**</u>

I think I slept pretty well. The meds the doctor prescribed seemed to help. Don't get me wrong, I still woke up several times but was able to go back to sleep. Doctors were in and said the final drainage tube was going to be removed today. They told me some of my levels from my blood tests were still not where they would like them but can be controlled by meds. If blood problems did not deteriorate, they said I could be discharged tomorrow or Friday. Good news!

During the day I met with a neurologist, had another swallow test and all was ok. PT was in and took me for a walk around the floor. I rode a recumbent bike to help strengthen my legs and talked about exercising at home to help me get back in shape.

Since I might be discharged tomorrow or Friday, we had to meet with my Case Manager who was scheduling my home care nurse for when I go home. When home I was to have a nurse, Physical Therapist (PT), and Occupational Therapist

(OT) and Speech Therapist (ST) to help me get back to somewhat of a normal living. pattern.

My Transplant Coordinator was in to begin talking about my discharge instructions and would finish when a final decision was made about the discharge.

This was a long day, and, in all honesty, it tired me out. If I have trouble sleeping tonight, at least I will be able to blame it on the excitement of knowing I will probably be going home in a day or two.

August 19

What a day this was. Everything pointed to me being discharged today. I slept pretty well; out of bed in my chair waiting for what I hoped was going to be my last round of them checking my vitals, drawing blood, x-rays, morning breathing tests, etc. The doctors were in and said I would be discharged later today.

Karen received a call from my Transplant Coordinator, and they were to meet at the outpatient pharmacy at 1pm to get my prescription drugs I would need since I was being discharged.

As you are aware, Karen has been staying at the Gift of Life Family **House and had to return to check** out because I was being discharged and heading back to Harrisburg.

Karen checked out of the Gift of Life Family House and was on her way back to the hospital to finish my discharge paperwork. She pulled into the parking garage, and I called her and said the discharge was not happening today. Some of my blood work was causing them concern. The tests that were way out of range were my electrolytes, WBC (White Blood Count), kidney function and hemoglobin.

I figured ok, this is just another bump in the road and nothing I will not be able to overcome. Besides, I think I have my room paid for through the end of the week.

August 20

I guess today will hopefully have less confusion than yesterday did. The day started just like yesterday. Karen checked out of the Gift of Life Family House (for the 2nd time), got partway to the hospital and received a call from me saying I would be a guest here at Temple until at least Monday. She had to get her room back again at the Gift of Life Family House. The doctors were still concerned about my blood tests. The same tests as yesterday were concerning to the team. Although we were both disappointed about not being discharged, we also know the importance of staying until everything is right. The last thing we want is to get home, have something happen and need to come back to Temple or another hospital.

Other than being told I wouldn't be going home until at least Monday; it was an uneventful day. I had the routine finger sticks, insulin shots and heparin shots. I would be remiss if I did not include the nurses checking on me, x-ray, breathing tests, blood work, etc.

August 21

Same routine as other mornings, not much activity on the weekends, things slow down and sometimes seem to go into slow motion. Bloodwork still not where they want it. Blood pressure still high and PT did not come around today, but they allowed Karen to walk with me. And it was another night of restless sleep. On the bright side, I did see a medical helicopter land on the heliport across the street.

August 22

Same routine as yesterday, didn't sleep well, out of bed waiting for the parade of people to start: breathing tests, x-ray, blood draw, finger prick, shots, meds, breakfast and wait for the doctors to arrive with their contingent of med students in tow.

Karen made it in time for the doctors' rounds, and we were pleased to hear my blood pressure and glucose were down and the blood count and kidney function were better today. Once again, the parting words of the doctors were "you will be discharged tomorrow." I think I will just wait until tomorrow to see if my discharge really happens.

PT was in today and we did walk the floor. I must admit I am not anywhere to the point where I could even think about walking any distance on my own. I will make this comparison to where I was after my first transplant and where I am now. Eight years ago, I walked into the hospital. I decided if I walked in, I could walk out. Well, I did it, but it wasn't the smartest thing I ever did and I will guarantee when it comes time for me to leave Temple, this time I will be pushed in a wheelchair to the exit.

This delay in my discharge is beginning to work on my Case Manager's nerves. She is trying to schedule a home health care nurse to come to the house, but she too keeps setting something up and then has to call them back and reschedule. I guess she will be working on scheduling tomorrow.

Here it is the day I have been waiting for… the day for my discharge. Just because I was going home, the morning routine has not changed. I didn't sleep well, out of bed waiting for the parade of people to start: breathing tests, x-ray, blood draw, finger prick, shots, meds, breakfast and wait for the doctors to arrive with their contingent of med students in tow.

Karen came to the hospital in time for the doctor's visit and to hear them say everything looked good, and they were going to complete the discharge paperwork.

Yea… now all we needed was the paperwork to be finished and meet with my Transplant Coordinator and finish the discharge instructions. Well, what could go wrong, I'm almost out the door!

Apparently, the transplant surgeon re-read the x-ray and saw what appeared to be fluid building around my transplanted lung. In the grand scheme of things, this is not good thing. He put the kibosh to me going home today. I probably will be spending another day or so here at Temple.

The doctor ordered another CT scan and then will be planning their next step, which will probably mean another drainage tube being re-inserted in my side and staying a few more days here at Temple.

Karen had checked out of the Gift of Life Family House for the third time and had to return to re-register for a few more days. It is a good thing they are flexible with their reservations. They did not come for me to take me for my CT scan until after 7pm.

I guess this whole thing of yes you are being discharged, no you're not thing, could have been annoying and I will admit, after a while, it was. But in all honesty, it was better having these issues, blood levels being out of whack and the fluid build-up around my lung here at the hospital rather than being at home and having to make a fast trip back to Temple. I was where I was supposed to be when all this happened. Someone upstairs was looking out for me.

Maybe I am learning to be a little more patient with things, especially things out of my control.

Let's just see what adventures tomorrow brings!

<u>August 24</u>

Today started out slow. Don't get me wrong everyone was in to do their respective jobs, but when the doctors were in things changed. The CT scan did confirm the fluid buildup around the lung and another chest tube was in my future. First, they had to do a Doppler Scan to make certain they place the drainage tube at the proper place. After the Doppler is done of the chest area the tube insertion will need to be scheduled.

I was wheeled into the procedure room a little after **11am** to have the Doppler done. They started scanning my arms and legs and I tried to tell them this wasn't what I was here for. The Doppler test was to get me ready to have a drainage tube inserted in my side. The technicians did stop to check their schedules to see if what they were doing was correct. According to them, it was and they continued. Now I was confused and annoyed. I was told I would get the procedure done and maybe have the tube inserted today.

I asked to see the doctor when I got back to my room. I needed to find out what was happening. Dr. Shenoy was as confused as I was and said he would find out. When he returned, he told me I had been scheduled for two Doppler tests today. One is my pre-discharge Doppler, the one I just had. They are checking to make certain when I am discharged I have no blood clots. This Doppler is normally done on the day of discharge. I don't think I am being discharged today, and, if I am, no one told me.

They eventually came for me around 4pm for my second Doppler and did the test and then did the tube insertion. They inserted this tube into an area between my ribs and into a sac where the fluid buildup is located. All this was being done while I am awake with only a numbing agent to take the edge off the procedure. I will say, I did not feel any pain only minor discomfort at times. Let the drainage begin and maybe I can get out of here.

August 25

Another day at Temple starting early with the usual cast of characters coming through my room... nurses, x-ray Technician, **phlebotomists**, you know the regulars I have been talking about for the past two weeks.

The doctors and/or team stopped in several times to check on the drainage and to see how I was feeling. I feel good after all of this running around.

After everything that has happened over the past week about me being discharged, Dr. Shenoy said "maybe you can go home Friday." I just shook my head, chuckled and told him I will believe it when I see it.

I was able to do physical therapy today and did several laps around the floor. I am still being very cautious as I walk, and I still tire rather quickly.

August 26

The start of another day, same routine, just maybe new faces. A nurse from Interventional Radiology came to check on the fluid draining from my lung. It appears I am not draining any fluid and this is a good thing. If the doctors sign off, he will return to remove the tube.

The doctors came in and asked how I was doing, I replied I felt fine. He rechecked the drainage tube and felt comfortable having the tube removed. One more x-ray was ordered. If it came back clear of fluid buildup and if Dr. Shigemura the transplant surgeon gave his blessing, he would begin the discharge process again. I was blessed and the discharge process began again.

While we waited, Karen met my transplant coordinator at the pharmacy, picked up my new supply of drugs, and I walked around the floor for one final **time with the** physical therapist. We go back to my room and wouldn't you know it, my surgical dressing covering my wound from my latest tube being taken out was leaking around the bandage. I thought this can't be happening. This isn't something that is going to keep me in the hospital for another day or so, is it? Fortunately, the bandage was not applied properly and after my transplant coordinator redressed the wound, we had no problem with leakage on our trip home.

They called for someone to take me to the exit. After my experience eight years ago, there was no way I was going to walk to the exit, and even though I did not want to ride in a wheelchair I was going to take advantage of this ride. In fact, I was taken right to our car that was parked in the parking garage.

Before we could head west on the PA Turnpike to Harrisburg, we needed to return to the Gift of Life Family house one final time so Karen could check-out for the fourth time on this trip. I waited in the car while she checked out and retrieved her belongings. While there I was asked to ring the "Chimes of Hope" which were erected to honor patients and their families who were able to celebrate milestones in their transplant journey. **I rang the Chimes of Hope for various reasons: having my transplant, thankful for my Donor, spending 16 days at TUH, Karen staying here at the Gift of Life Family House, and now heading home.** These are milestones needing to be celebrated.

The trip heading west on the PA Turnpike was long and uneventful. It was tiring for me, and sleeping in my own bed with someone I love felt really great. I slept well, probably the best I have slept since before I went to Temple on August 9th.

Before I move on, I must give a shout out to a few people. Well, it is really too many people for me to thank individually. I can't think of anyone that would not need complemented while I was a patient at Temple University Hospital from August 9th - August 26th.

Starting with the people in the Admissions Office who waited until I arrived to make sure all the paperwork was in order, the technicians and nurses in pre-op who made certain we were comfortable while I waited for the transplant to begin, and the transplant team who assisted the doctors who performed the transplant. While I am thanking people who were in the OR, a big shoutout goes to the surgeon who gave me a 'third' chance at life, Dr. Norih Shigemura.

Thanks to all the nurses and staff in the ICU and on the Stepdown Unit. I know the jobs that you were doing were difficult, especially being shorthanded and doing all this during a pandemic. Thank you for what you did not only for me but for all the patients you were charged with taking care of.

Thanks to Dr. Nathan Marchetti and Dr. Kartik Shenoy who were the attending doctors during my stay at Temple. They did their best to keep me calm during my period of yes you will be discharged, no you won't be discharged part of my stay. Thanks for not allowing me to leave until I was ready to go.

Thank you to Dr. Francis Cordova, my Transplant Pulmonologist and his team who have been on this journey with me from the very beginning. They have guided me and kept me healthy not only through one transplant but now two of them. I know this may not have been easy, but thank you for your support.

Temple University Hospital should be proud of each and every one of you!

<u>**August 27 – 29**</u>

Just because I am home from the hospital, my transplant journey is not over by any stretch of anyone's imagination. Tomorrow my post-transplant recovery continues at home…

These three days were mainly R & R (Rest and Recuperation) for both Karen and me; we both slept well each night and woke up semi-refreshed.

On the 27th Karen redressed my wound that had been seeping fluid since shortly before I came home. The seepage had stopped and Karen only needed a band aid to cover the last wound.

My first trip out of house was to the barber shop for a shave and a haircut, and you know it only cost two bits…

Home Health Care stopped by to do an evaluation and to determine what help I may need to continue recovery. Arrangements were made to have a Nurse, Physical Therapist (PT), Occupational Therapist (PT) and Speech Therapist (ST).

August 30 – September 13

Another good night's sleep. It's amazing what being home can do for your recovery. I had to get up early to have blood drawn for weekly testing. It seems like a long time since someone drew blood, but it's only been a few days… four days to be exact. I had to get home to meet with the Home Health Care administrator to set up a visitation schedule for me; besides, I had nowhere else to go.

First a nurse was to come and give me a physical; I guess to establish a baseline of sorts for their records. PT came to start me on an in-home exercise program to do two times a day; by no means was it difficult for me to do.

The OT was next at the door. She was here to make certain that I could do normal daily chores without doing harm to myself. She found I had no difficulty with any of her exercises. This was the first and last visit for her.

ST came to make certain was not having any issues with my speech and I wasn't. She gave me some breathing exercises to help strengthen **muscles** used in speech. She practiced the exercises with me and said she didn't think I needed her services and would not be coming back.

This was my first week of home visitation with my Home Health Care representatives. Four visits and the Nurse and PT are the only two who will return.

The 3rd **of September** saw my first post-transplant doctor visit, and it was a good one. I had an x-ray. It showed a little fluid buildup around the transplanted lung, but it wasn't concerning at this time. Half of the staples were removed, and the rest would be removed at the next appointment. I asked about removing the port from my photopheresis study and was told it was too early. I asked about getting my COVID-19 vaccine booster and was told to get it 90 days after transplant. The only concern I had was I was losing weight. Dr. Cordova sent a note to the dietician to contact me to discuss my weight loss **and I was to** return in two weeks for my next appointment.

During those two weeks I had two sessions with the PT to do some leg strengthening exercises and talked to the nurse once on the telephone. PT is happy with the progress I have made with the exercises and said I should soon be released. The nurse suggests I do one more session and I agreed.

During this two-week period, I also tried to get back into some sort of routine, like I had before my transplant in

August. I say a routine, but it is more like just having some sort of a schedule to follow. I wanted to become part of Zoom meetings which I was part of before, i.e., support groups, anything but doctors' appointments. I met with my dermatologist to make certain I did not have any spots needing to be checked further. This appointment was scheduled prior to my transplant, but it is something the doctors want to make certain we do on a regular schedule.

September 14 - 26

I had an appointment at Temple today and it too went well. I had a PFT, x-ray and blood draw, and all were good. We talked about the benefit of pulmonary rehab vs Home Health Care, and it was agreed pulmonary rehab would benefit me more. I got a script so I could start pulmonary rehab at PSHMC. Some of my meds were changed for the first time since I came home. I was to return for my next appointment in about two weeks.

Along with the weekly blood draws we had numerous Zoom meetings with various support groups and the Pulmonary Fibrosis Foundation. We also managed to get out for a few car rides, and, of course, we had to pick-up the groceries we ordered.

On the 15th I had my last PT session. It was uneventful. Now all I needed was the nurse and the administrator to come for one final review. PT showed up as expected, but the nurse and administrator didn't show up to finish the paperwork.

Finally, on the 21st everybody showed up when they were supposed to, the paperwork was signed, and I was now finished with Home Health Care. I am certain they provide a good service and are needed in the community, but it wasn't meant for me.

On the 22nd as we have done in past years to celebrate my "8th lungaversary," we provided a meal for the guests staying at the Gift of Life Family House. It was not a home cooked meal. We weren't there to prepare it, but it was home cooked from the heart. As I have said the past couple of years... maybe next year!

September 27 – September 30

Today I had an appointment, pft's, and met with Dr. Cordova. Pft's were good and while my blood pressure was down to almost normal range, now my pulse rate goes up. Probably a result of some of my drugs. Again, we need to adjust some meds.

The new concern is my recent loss of weight. When I left the hospital, my weight was just about what it was pre-transplant at 195 pounds. Since I was released earlier this month, I have lost about 15 pounds. Now I have a dietician working with me to make certain I am eating the right foods. I need to stop losing weight and put some of the lost weight back on. This is a switch, usually they are telling us to lose weight and not gain it. I see some Wendy's chocolate Frosty's in my future!

I am still trying to get my port removed, again I was told after my next visit.

On the 28th I began my PR (Pulmonary Rehab). I will be doing PR twice a week for 13 weeks and then I will start exercising on my own at the gym. I have each rehab session scheduled, and I will be at the PR lab each Tuesday and

Thursday. After all, I have made promises to take extra good care of these two gifts I have received.

My next appointment at Temple is on October 15th.

October 15

I met with Dr. Cordova today. He said it was okay to get my third shot of the Moderna at the 90-day anniversary of my transplant. This will be in about a month. For the most part my bloodwork was good but a little concerned about the low WBC.

I mentioned to Dr. Cordova that since the transplant I have been a little unstable when I walk. If you have heard the phrase "walking like a drunken sailor," well, that's me for sure. Dr. Cordova did a few in-office tests like walking a straight line, close your eyes and touch your nose with your finger, those types of tests. Well, it's safe to say I didn't do well on those basic tests. He wanted me to meet with a neurologist and have an MRI of the brain completed. We will talk more about the results at next month's appointment.

Pulmonary Rehab is going well and glad it was suggested I do it. I think my pulmonary rehab sessions will end sometime in December. This is just another way that I am staying active and at least getting some exercise.

November 15

Met with Dr. Cordova and went over the bloodwork, pft's, echo and MRI. MRI shows abnormal small chronic hemorrhage on the right front lobe. Hopefully what they are seeing is something which comes with age and not a sign of a small stroke…

I met with my cardiologist, had an ekg completed, and all is well with the heart. At least I finally get a report with a Gold Star on it.

I had my third COVID -19 vaccine booster shot earlier this month. I asked about how long we should wait to see if this shot had any effect on any antibodies being built up to fend off the virus. He gave me a script to get tested one month after my third shot. I will have this test done before my next appointment which is December 13th.

December 13

Another good meeting with Dr. Cordova. My pft's were a little lower, but he was not concerned. Went over my med list and no changes. This doesn't happen often, at least not to me. My 14-week pulmonary rehab sessions have ended, I graduated and they gave me a diploma I could hang on my wall. The following week I will start going to the gym two or three times a week for exercise.

I had my blood tested for antibodies earlier this week. Good news, the test came back positive with antibodies. I don't know how long they will last, but I am sure they will do the job while they are in this body of mine.

Dr. Cordova wants me to have my PCP check for a groin hernia when I see him next month and to have a 12 lead ekg and a blood test for B12/folate, all before my next appointment in January.

I thought Christmas 2020 was a little weird, I mean everything was cancelled. We basically had Christmas via Zoom. This year feels a little weird also. I mean with COVID-19 still hanging around and Karen and I being in the senior age bracket, and me being immuno suppressed, we really were between a rock and a hard place. We wanted to have our families together, but we wanted to make sure everyone was safe and COVID-19 free.

Our dilemma was this: we have four kids and their families. Three families are planning to come home for a total of 14 people. One family had three members who had returned from a Mexican vacation the week before; another family had one coming home from the military on leave; another family member was coming home from a wrestling tournament in Colorado; and finally, the remaining family coming from out of state had one who was a high school student and her sister was coming home from college. Everyone, in one way or another, could easily have been in contact with someone who was carrying the virus.

Every one of us has been vaccinated and a couple of us have anti-bodies built up. Karen and I have been careful during this pandemic; we do what we can to avoid crowds and be safe. We want to have the family together for Christmas, but we want everyone to be safe. Our choices are this… we cancel Christmas and become the Scrooge of the family, or we can do it via Zoom like we did last year, or everyone comes to the house, and we will let whatever happens happen, or we can all take the test before the 25th and hope everyone shows up negative.

We had our family Zoom meeting the Sunday prior to Christmas. We expressed our concerns and discussed the options we came up with. All agreed that the test was the best option. We were happy and excited that everyone's test came back negative, and we were able to be together to celebrate Christmas.

As this month comes to a close, so does 2021. This year has been different for us. This entire year has included some type of COVID-19 protocol, whether it be a lockdown of some sort, mask usage, COVID-19 vaccines, crowded hospitals, a death toll that keeps rising, bare shelves at the grocery store or other things too numerous to mention. Things are very different than most of us would like to see.

Each of us, no matter how low our spirits are or have been this year can certainly find something positive that we can be thankful for in 2021! For me, I am thankful for the Gift of Life that I received on August 10th. I received the right lung of a 31-year-old man who died too early. That's what I am thankful for, and I hope you all had a Merry Christmas!

<u>**2022**</u>

January - Happy New Year Everyone. I had my pork and sauerkraut today and now I should have good luck for the rest of the year. Other than blood tests and pft's, I have no other appointments at Temple until the 24th.

Finally, I am having the port that I had inserted in my chest back in May 2020 removed. It was to be removed after my post -transplant office visit, which technically it was, but not soon enough. This surgery was completed in less than 15 minutes, 30 if you count the time spent in the waiting room on January 24th.

My pft's, they were stable; of course, I was hoping for some sort of increase in my numbers.

I met with Dr. Cordova, and he said I could now have my blood work done every other week. This is due to my bloodwork stabilizing.

Nothing to be concerned about, and both lungs are strong. As Karen likes to say, *"the kids are playing nice together in the sandbox!"* Maybe, this would be a good book title?

My next appointment at Temple will be in three months. I guess it is good that I am able to begin 2022 the same way I left 2021… on a positive note.

As I said seven years ago, I think it is now time for me to discontinue my writing. I see no value at this time to put more words on paper just to take up space. Okay, this brings me to the point where I can say… and as they say, the rest is going to be history!

For details of my journey from January 2009 to December 2014 you might want to read or re-read my first book titled… *New Mountains to Climb"* which is still available on Amazon.

<u>**Epilogue**</u>

Although I have halted writing about my day-to-day journey, I want to share some of the things I have learned during the past eight or nine years.

<u>**Writing to your Donor Family**</u>

Since my transplant, I have often been asked about writing to my Donor Family. My answer has always been this. You and only you know if it is the right thing for you to do and when to write this letter. I will say from my perspective that this is one of the most difficult letters I have ever written. This is the second time I wrote an initial letter to my donor family. Remember, I wrote a letter back in 2014 after I had my first transplant. Writing the second time was not any easier.

Some individuals think a letter is not necessary; others say they can't find the right words to put down on paper; and then there are people who think they should write to the family as soon as possible.

I believe my advice would be this... don't write too soon. Remember the family that you are writing to just lost a loved one and the family may still be grieving the loss. Many of the transplant hospitals will provide you information as to how you should properly write this letter. Ask the social worker you might be working with for help. They will gladly help you and then send the letter to the family for you.

If you do send this letter, please keep in mind there is no guarantee the family will respond back to you.

I have included two letters I wrote to my Donor Families to use as examples.

When completed I forwarded them to the Donate Life organization in Philadelphia who in turn forward the letters to the respective donor families. I keep hoping each time I go to the mailbox I will find a letter from my donors' family. I have been told it is not unusual not to hear from them; sometimes it takes a while for the family to feel comfortable to send a response; and it is possible I will never get that letter I keep hoping for.

This is a letter I wrote to my donor family after my first transplant.

November 27, 2014

> **Dear Donor Family,**
>
> *Hi it's me again, Jim! It has been nine months since I last wrote and I continue to count my blessings each day.*
>
> *I felt that this might be a good time for me to write and tell you how thankful I have been since I received the precious gift from your loved one. I continue to struggle finding the right words to say to you and your family. I would like you to know that your loved one and your family are in my thoughts and prayers every day. I know I will never be able to thank you enough for giving me a second chance at life.*
>
> *The doctors continue to be quite pleased with my recovery and I feel stronger every day. I am not*

out running any distances yet, but I do try to keep active. Since the weather has changed, I have become a mall walker and walk on a regular basis and most days I walk 2 – 3 miles if not farther.

I had set a few goals for myself for this year; some which I thought would be doable for me. I wanted to mow my own lawn, which I did. My grandson was doing a great job, but there was something about the satisfaction of doing it on my own.

Since my wife had gotten me a gift certificate for a couple of golf lessons, I wanted to do some golfing this year, but I quickly found out that I was not going to be able to accomplish that goal. When I tried to swing a golf club it became apparent that the muscles in my side have not healed enough to let me go out on the golf course to play at this time. Oh well I will try for next year.

Another goal was to be able to walk a mile in 15 minutes. Although I walk several miles a day, this goal has eluded me. It takes me about 16 or 17 minutes to do this so I still have some work to do.

I know those goals that I have set for myself seem small in comparison to what some others are facing; I keep remembering that fourteen months ago I would not have been able to do any of those goals or many other things that my wife and I have been able to do without the gift that I received from your loved one.

I continue hoping that one day, when the time is right, we will have the opportunity to meet so that I can personally say thank you to you and your family.

Your loved one continues to live through me and that with his help I am trying to live my life in a way that would make you proud.

I continue to hope that life treats your family to nothing but happiness and prosperity. If there is anything you would like to know about or from me, please feel free to contact me.

Again, I just want to say thank from the bottom of my heart.

This second letter I wrote to my Donor Family after my second transplant and sent it to them after six months. I haven't had a response from them, and I don't know if I will.

February 10, 2022

Dear Family,

My name is Jim, and I am the 72-year-old retired male who received a precious gift from your loved one. I know of no words that can truly express my feelings for your family; it takes a special kind of person to make such a sacrifice in their time of grief. I would like you to know you and your family are in my thoughts and prayers every day. I know I will never be able to thank you enough for giving me a third chance at life.

In 2009 I was diagnosed with pulmonary fibrosis and on September 22, 2013 I received a gift of a left lung from another unselfish donor. This gave me a second chance at life. In 2019 I started going through chronic rejection and on August 10th, 2021 I received another special gift that saved my life again. I promise I will take care of this gift I received, a gift that gave me a third chance at life. Each night before I go to sleep and each morning before I get out of bed, I take a moment to reflect on my lungs steadily pumping life sustaining oxygen through my body. The lung is alive and healthy and has created in me a new appreciation for life.

I thought you might like to know the doctors say everything is progressing extremely well. I have had no major problems and the right lung is functioning extremely well. As I write this letter, almost six months after my transplant, I want you to know that I would have written sooner, but I wanted to make certain everything was working out so I could show you what has been accomplished by your family's loved one's decision to donate.

I am aware the lung I received is not mine. It belonged to the kind of person all of us should want to be. Maybe it is my imagination but since receiving my new lung, I feel a peace I haven't felt before.

I appreciate the simple things now, much more than before. I look forward every morning to seeing my loving wife and caregiver, Karen. Each day gives me a new thrill because each day is a gift from you and from GOD.

My hope is one day we will meet so I can personally say thank you. If or when that does happen, I will likely be at a loss for words. You gave me life; you gave me peace and you gave me a profound sense of gratitude and understanding. I am a new person and I hope in your grief it helps to know a part of your loved one is alive in me and with his help I am trying to live my life in a way that would make you proud.

My wife and I would also like to say how sorry we are for your loss. It is nice to know there are such special people in this world who care about other people so much.

Saying thank you just doesn't seem like enough when what somebody does is basically save your life. I sincerely hope life treats your family to nothing but happiness and prosperity. If there is anything you would like to know about or from me, please feel free to contact me.

Again, I just want to say thank you from the bottom of my heart!

These letters were not easy to write, but I personally felt the need to do them. I will continue to write to my new Donor Family. If for no other reason, I will let them know the GIFT I received is being taken care of.

<u>**Pulmonary Rehabilitation**</u>

Throughout my book I have been stressing the need for us to stay healthy, both pre- and post-transplant. One way is to have your doctor sign you up (write you a script) for pulmonary rehab. I have done several sessions, and, most recently, I had been going twice a week. After those sessions ended, I started going to the gym two or three times a week.

According to the Pulmonary Fibrosis Foundation, pulmonary rehabilitation (PR) is a structured exercise program designed for people living with chronic lung diseases like pulmonary fibrosis (PF). Pulmonary rehabilitation includes exercise training; breathing exercises; anxiety, stress, and depression management; nutritional counseling; education; and more.

People with idiopathic pulmonary fibrosis (IPF) and other types of PF can experience increasing shortness of breath and cough. These symptoms may lead to a progressive decline in physical activities and social isolation, and worsening breathlessness, fatigue, and mood disorders including depression and anxiety. Pulmonary rehabilitation has been found to improve physical function, breathlessness (dyspnea), mood, and quality of life in people with IPF and other types of PF.

<u>**Caregivers**</u>

I can't say enough about caregivers, especially <u>**my**</u> caregiver who just happens to be my wife and best friend. I am sure if you would ask her, she would say this just happens to be part of the marriage contract; I guess she is looking at the part referring to "in sickness and in health." Karen has been by my side at every test and doctor's appointment I have had since my journey with pulmonary fibrosis began. She was with me when I was going through my difficult times during my journey. She was the one sitting in the waiting room as I was going through various procedures during my transplant evaluations. She was the one who took the phone call from Temple on that Sunday morning telling us they had a lung for me and she was the one who waited anxiously for word about how my surgery was progressing. Her smiling face was the first one I saw when I woke up in the ICU. She has been my nurse, my cheerleader, my go-fer, my sounding board, my chauffer, my biggest supporter, and as she is fond of saying, she has been my drill sergeant throughout this journey. In my mind, after the role of the transplant surgeon, the caregiver has the most important role in your recovery!

Life After Transplant

You have just had a major surgery for which you will likely enjoy an improved quality of life. Most patients who have a transplant breathe better, increase their activity, and can discontinue supplemental oxygen. Maybe you will go back to work and travel. But even when surgery results are positive, life after a transplant has its own challenges. To maintain the best possible health and reduce the chance of complications, you'll need to follow your transplant team's instructions throughout your life. Having a transplant means you have made a lifetime commitment to taking care of the gift you received.

Once you've left the hospital, your early recovery process continues at home. You should have at least one caregiver available so that someone can be with you 24 hours a day for the first several weeks after surgery. Most lung transplant programs caution against driving in the early recovery period to avoid strain on the incision site from turning the steering wheel. Many programs caution against lifting more than five pounds for similar reasons. They don't want you to put pressure on the incision. You should avoid crowds, especially with COVID and flu season rearing their ugly heads. Wearing a mask is always a good idea. You might want to restrict visitors to your home while you're recovering. Frequent hand washing is an important way to prevent the spread of infection. Contact your care team if you have any of the following problems: a redness or swelling of the incision, blood or other fluid leaking from the incision, pain around the incision that gets worse, fever or shortness of breath or trouble breathing. These are just some of the things that will be strongly suggested that you should do.

Encouraging survival stats: Approximately 89% of lung transplant patients survive at least one year after their surgery. After three years, approximately 74% of individuals receiving lung transplants are still alive. Many factors contribute to survival post-transplant, including age, disease type, severity of illness at the time of transplant, and procedure type. Survival rates have continued to improve over recent years.

Source: Organ Procurement and Transplantation Network and Scientific Registry of Transplant Recipients 2018 Annual Data Report

Support Groups

I sincerely believe that families and friends should be included under the heading of support groups. Each in their own unique ways are a benefit, not only to the patient, but also the caregiver. Both should be included in this group.

Your immediate family should be your first line of support and next come your close friends.

Having the support of your entire family and/or friends is probably a pipe dream for most patients, especially when it comes to a disease like pulmonary fibrosis. Heck, this is a disease we never heard of, so why should we expect them to know what we are talking about!

Having a few people in your life support you, educate themselves about your condition, learn about the medical choices you have to make and actively take a role in caregiving for you is a major blessing. I'm lucky to have a handful of these people in my life who understand my disease. Some have been there all along, and some finally understand that there was a difference between who you are and what you have.

Without all of the offers of help and support coming our way since this journey began, and, especially since my transplant, this trip could have been much more difficult for both Karen and me. Just receiving a phone call to say hi or to see if we needed anything has meant so much to both of us.

They are the ones who will always be there for you, no matter what is going on.

If you are not part of a support group, find one to get involved with. Some hospitals, especially transplant hospitals, have meetings you can attend. Where else can you go and be surrounded by people who are going through the same experiences? There you can talk about how you feel, get answers to questions you have (and GOD knows you have many questions about this disease) from people who probably have or had some of the same questions you have. The people who attend were once in the same place you are currently in: confused and scared. Most transplant centers, if not all of them, want you, as a patient and caregiver, to attend these meetings.

Connecting with others facing similar experiences can improve emotional well-being and have a positive impact on the health of people who are living with pulmonary fibrosis.

A support group can also be a valuable source of encouragement and inspiration for patients, caregivers, family members, and friends.

<u>Humor</u>

I believe if you have read my story, you will note my attempt at humor being infused with seriousness throughout this document. Early on I found out what they have said about humor being a great medicine to be very true. Please don't think I take, or anybody should take, this deadly disease lightly. I chose very early on to not let this disease beat me, and maybe you can say I am laughing in the face of this disease, but it is my way of dealing with pulmonary fibrosis. I have a disease I didn't ask for, and I chose the path I am now following, it is just I choose not to cry about what happened, but rather smile, laugh and make the best of situation that has changed my life and changed the lives of those closest to me.

Remember the saying: if you laugh, the whole world laughs with you, and if you cry, you cry alone!

It is your choice as to how you proceed on your own journey.

Faith

This is probably the part of my story I shouldn't be talking about, only because of everyone's different take on religion, but for me it was a big part of my journey.

I have always believed in GOD. Have I waivered at times? Absolutely I have! In my youth, dealing with the death of loved ones, during and after my Vietnam experience, and especially after I was diagnosed with pulmonary fibrosis, my faith probably waivered again. To be honest, each of these experiences, especially the IPF and transplant experience, has probably renewed my faith and made it stronger.

I have prayed for guidance as I traveled the road toward transplant; I have prayed for renewed healing strength for myself; I have prayed for the guidance and expertise of the medical staff as they led me down the road toward transplant and for the steady hands of the surgical team who successfully completed my transplants.

Does prayer work? I absolutely believe it does! I have said my recovery is in the hands of GOD and the excellent medical staff looking after my care and recovery.

The following is something I wrote several years ago, and as I now approach my nine year "lungaversary" for my first transplant and now toward my "one-year lungaversary" for my second transplant, I feel this is as pertinent now as it was then… and maybe, just maybe, it will serve as a bridge to the next portion of my journey.

On our way to church, Karen and I were discussing transplants and how their outcomes affect not only patients but also the caregivers. She asked me if I was satisfied with my outcome and if I had any regrets.

Maybe it was because I wasn't quite awake yet or maybe I might be able to blame it on not having had my first cup of coffee, but for a moment I was at a loss for words and this is something that does not happened to me, especially when it comes to the subject of lung transplantation, but I must admit, the words did not flow as quickly as I would have liked.

After a few moments of silent reflection, I think I responded by saying I am probably one of the luckiest people in the world and had <u>no regrets</u> about answering this call back in September 2013. I know how blessed I have been to have received the call many still wait for each day. Each night before I go to bed and each morning, I thank GOD and my Donor family for the Second Chance at Life I received, and to be able to talk to others about this disease we have been afflicted with.

I know there are some days I get up and wonder when I will feel normal again and then I quickly realize I do feel normal; what I am experiencing is "my new normal" we all talk about and to be honest, I wouldn't trade this feeling for the world.

Certainly, I would like to hike again or be able to exert myself the way I did before I was diagnosed with I.P.F., but this is not my normal now and I need to adapt to doing things at a slightly different pace than what I once did.

I have no regrets and I am quite satisfied about undergoing a single lung transplant and the outcome. I am still me; I still do many of the things I used to do; I am still loved by my family and friends and each day I still thank GOD and my Donor family for this Second Chance I received.

As I have said many times to people, having the transplant sure beats the alternative.

Gift of Life Family House

Throughout my IPF and transplant journey the Gift of Life Family House had become an important part of my adventure. Several of them I had mentioned in this book. The Gift of Life Family House is similar to the Ronald McDonald House in Hershey, PA and I believe throughout the USA. This house is used for patients and families who are in town for doctors' appointments at one of the six area transplant hospitals in Philadelphia. The Gift of Life Family House became a home away from home for us after long days of testing at Temple. We were able to go back to the Gift of Life Family House and relax, get a hot meal, and talk to others who were experiencing the same issues as we were. It gave us someone to talk to and gain more information pertaining to this journey we were on. Some of the people were there because they were going through the same evaluations I was. Some people had had transplants and were in town for follow-up appointments. Some were families who were there because they had someone in the hospital who had received a transplant, and there were people at the Gift of Life Family House who were there waiting for an organ to become available so they could receive a transplant and a second chance at life and in my case a third chance. If you are being seen at one of the Philadelphia hospitals, check them out. They are welcoming and offer you a home away from home.

Donor and Donor Families

I would be remiss if I did not mention our donors and their families. If it were not for the donors, and their families abiding by their wishes, those of us who have had a transplant, might not be here and I would not have had the opportunity to share parts of my journey with you.

Some families say that being able to donate their loved one's organs is the one silver lining to come out of a nightmarish personal storm.
 There's no way around it: Funerals are difficult. Yet a final gift can save lives and bring healing to other families. Something positive can come out of the pain.
 Organ donation offers one-person incredible power to change lives.
 Organ donation can help surviving family members make sense of their loss. Following a donation, sometimes we remain in contact with the organ donors' family and provide continued support.

Sometimes, family members are motivated by the prospect that "something positive could come out of their loss," that "someone else would have a better life," and that, in a way, "their family member lives on." This idea of paying life forward, and having something beautiful come out of their tragedy, is certainly compelling. It can be something encouraging to cling to in those first difficult days, months, even years.

None of us likes to think about our loved ones dying, much less to consider our own death. Yet, we tend to think giving the gift of life is more about life than death.

Even so, it's inevitable that each of us will die at some point, so it's really important that we make this very personal decision and share our wishes with our family members. If we don't talk about it, or don't document our wishes, we have either intentionally—or unintentionally—given the responsibility to our family to make the decision on our behalf. Our experience shows family members would rather not be in that position.

When we make the choice ourselves, and document it, we spare our family members from being burdened with one more emotional decision at a time when they'll likely be overwhelmed.

Many times, people say the reason they've not signed up to be a donor is because they've (wrongly) assumed that they are either too old or they have a certain medical condition that makes them ineligible. The truth is, there are absolutely no age restrictions to become an organ donor—and each donor's medical condition is carefully evaluated at the time of donation. Everyone is encouraged to sign-up to become an organ donor, no matter your age or medical history.

What I have been trying to say in the last two pages is pretty well summed up in the following quote by UNOS: *"Without the organ donor, there is no story, no hope, no transplant. But when there is an organ donor,* life *springs from death, sorrow turns to hope and a terrible loss becomes a gift."*

<u>A word of advice...</u>

No matter where you are on this journey, stay off the Internet, and if you can't stay off, don't believe everything you read is necessarily the truth and applies to your case. You must keep in mind this is where some well-meaning people who are on or have been on this journey come together to share their experiences and offer advice as to what may have worked them, and this is just what it is, their experiences.

This disease affects each of us differently, and, as you know, there is no cookie cutter cure for IPF. How I am being treated is probably not the same way you are going to be treated. Listen to your doctors, not some well-meaning person who believes his or her treatment is better or worse than what your doctor is prescribing.

Listen to what your doctor is telling you. He or she is the expert. After all, this is why he or she is being paid the big bucks. If there is something wrong with you, please don't call me or any other patient for advice. Call your doctor. He or she is the one who is going to be able to help you. All I am going to do is tell you to call your doctor.

Each time I talk to a group or an individual about pulmonary fibrosis, I qualify what I am about to tell them is how this journey or this disease has affected me and not necessarily how it is going to affect them or anybody else.

Here are three organizations I use quite often to get or verify information about this disease: the Pulmonary Fibrosis Foundation can be reached at www.pulmonaryfibrosis.org, the Wescoe Foundation for Pulmonary Fibrosis can be reached at wescoefoundationforpulmonaryfibrosis.org and the American Lung Association can be reached at lung@.org

All other thoughts and feelings...

I really didn't know where to put this, so I made it its own heading.

The journey that we have been on has not always given us a warm and fuzzy feeling. Sometimes what we hear is downright depressing, especially when we hear of the death of someone who also has been on this very same journey that we are on. I can count almost 20 individuals who have passed away since I started this journey in 2009.

During the Lenten period of 2021 I was challenged by our minister to write a short article about the people we had met on our "Journey to Jerusalem" leading up to our Easter celebration.

I must admit I struggled finding just one person to write about. The reason why I struggled was I chose to write about someone I had met on my journey with pulmonary fibrosis. There were many people I could have written about but ultimately in my first writing I chose my donor and his family. As you continue reading you will see why I struggled. The first writing is what a wrote for my Lenten challenge. The second is what I could have written about but thought it might be a little long for our church publication.

Read on and I hope you might see why I struggled…

<u>The People we meet… Part I</u>

Many of you are aware I was the recipient of a single lung transplant in 2013 and I am currently waiting for a second transplant. This is not about my journey per se, but rather people I never knew existed until the day of my transplant. I was very fortunate to have met them on the road to Jerusalem.

I knew somewhere this person existed, but our paths had never crossed. I guess it could have been possible we bumped into each other somewhere, but I doubt it.

I knew this person would have a family, but I had never met them either.

Everything changed on a beautiful sunny, Sunday morning in September. We were getting ready to leave for church and we received the call we had been waiting for… on September 22nd, 2013, a lung had become available for me!

Needless to say, I didn't meet this man in the usual way… no handshake or hug and no words of greeting. In fact, I never had the chance to hear his voice. In the beginning all I knew about him was he was a 36-year-old man who died too early in life. He was the man who gave me hope!

I wrote to his family hoping against hope I might get a return letter from them. I knew while I was celebrating a successful transplant, somewhere there was a family mourning the loss of someone very close to them.

I wrote to the family knowing I may never hear from them, but I needed to let them know the Gift I received from their loved one was being well taken care of and my recovery was going well. I told the family when and if the time was right for them and they would like to meet, I would be willing. I needed to show them the Gift I received from him was allowing me to breathe again.

Four years later, on another trip to Jerusalem, I met a family I had never met. They told me they knew me because I had written letters to their family telling them the lung I received in my transplant came from a family member. This was the family of my donor and they were finally ready to meet with me, and now I know the name of my donor and his name is **Juan**.

I knew each of us grieve in our own ways and it took his family a little longer than some, but I was glad I had this opportunity to meet and get to know each other better.

It took almost four years, but this trip to Jerusalem came to an end in a conference room in Alexandria, VA where Karen and I had the opportunity to learn more about Juan and his family. We met his mother, sister, daughter and granddaughter on the road to Jerusalem.

I am so blessed by my donor and his family and I am forever grateful. I found out Juan was a caring, selfless and loving person. They told me in their eyes he was a hero. Juan's last wish was to donate his organs so others may have a chance to live. At the time we met, the organs Juan donated were living on in five people including me.

In another time and place I would have been proud to call Juan my friend. Now I can only hope some of the traits he had will have rubbed off on me.

As they say, hindsight is 20/20, and I guess in this case it might be true. I think this is what I would have liked to have written!

<u>The People we meet… Part 2</u>

Previously I had written about a man I had never met, at least in a normal way. Of course, Juan would be at the top of my list. I met **Juan** on my journey on the road to Jerusalem, a man who has saved my life and the lives of at least four other individuals. Although I have had the opportunity to thank his family for the gift of life I received, someday, in another dimension, I hope to have the opportunity to say thank you to Juan.

Back in 2009 I was diagnosed with Pulmonary Fibrosis and at this time I started another journey on the road to Jerusalem. Over the course of my life, I have met many people, some have turned out to be not so nice, some have been just plain interesting, but most have turned out to be real friends.

Many of the people who turned out to be real friends had the same disease as me. I met many of them early on while I was trying to understand this disease and wondering just how this disease is going to affect not only my life but also those people around me.

Ed H. was the person who had the most influence on my decision to move forward toward transplant. I guess you might say we were "Support Group" friends. I will admit we never had much contact with each other except at support group meetings; but there he inspired me. Ed seemed always to be in a positive state of mind. Sadly, after a long struggle with issues both pre- and post-transplant he found peace and has gained his wings. Breathe easy my friend! Someday in another dimension I hope we will be able to meet again. At his memorial service, his wife whispered to me: "Don't let the negative outcome of his experiences affect my decision!" Those are words I will always remember.

On this very same journey, sitting at our table at a seminar about PF was **Maureen M.**, a very quiet and reserved person. Maureen did not speak much. Of course, none of us did because we were there to learn about this disease and get as much factual information about a disease none of us had ever heard of. Later on, our paths crossed again. While still on my journey to Jerusalem I met Maureen and her husband eating breakfast at the Gift of Life Family House in Philadelphia. Maureen had a single lung transplant about a month before I did. Once again, our paths crossed on my journey to Jerusalem. Sadly, Maureen gained her wings and is now at peace, breathing easily like she once did.

Joe L. Jobie, as he was known to his family, was the second person I met on this journey to Jerusalem. We were checking into the Gift of Life Family House for my transplant evaluation processing the next morning, and they were checking in to do the same thing. You might say the two of us have been on this journey together. He was a bit worse than I was and was transplanted prior to me. Joe developed problems and fought the good fight up to the very end, and, he, too, is wearing his wings and breathing easy.

Evie B. was a ball of fire and determined she was going to beat this disease. Evie was a smallish type person, and, thus, it would take a smaller set of lungs to fit in her chest cavity. She was determined she was going to be one of the people who would get those special lungs. She got the call on a wintry night, and she and her husband made the long trip to the hospital only to find out the donor's family decided not to donate his/her organs. Her wait continued, and she fought Pulmonary fibrosis to the very end. Evie is now sleeping with the angels. Breathe easy my friend!

Carl L. was our resident drummer in our support group. Carl is another person who left us too soon. He fought this disease like a true warrior to the bitter end. I don't think Carl would admit it, but you could see in his face the struggle he was fighting inside his body. Carl is now keeping the "backbeat" for the great band in heaven. Breathe easy my friend!

Paul H. Paul was in my training class of PFF Ambassadors learning about the PFF and how to share our experiences with others. Paul was from Washington State and spread the word about this dreaded disease to anyone who would listen. Paul spoke to groups and even started a PF Support in his home area. Paul left us too soon. Although Paul was a transplant survivor, he was fighting several battles at the end. Paul was hospitalized with COVID-19 and pneumonia. In the end he could not win the battle with COVID-19. Breathe easy my friend!

Fred W. would be the comedian in the group. He always had something to say to put a smile on your face or make you laugh. I met Fred, shortly after he was diagnosed with PF, and we talked multiple times about my transplant journey. Fred had his transplant and was doing well and then was diagnosed with cancer. Fred was fighting the battle on two fronts. One front was IPF and the other was cancer. Unfortunately, he lost his battle with another ugly disease… Cancer. Rest easy my friend!

Frank P. was our resident fireman in the group, just in case a blaze would break out for some unforeseen reason. I met Frank at a PFF meeting and then later on at a PFF Ambassador training session. Frank was not only a friend of mine but also a friend to many in the Pulmonary Fibrosis community. Frank was always willing to share his story with others. Rest in peace my friend.

These are not the only people I met on the road to Jerusalem. I could include without difficulty **Rafe' S., Dick C., Joe P., Glenda R., John M., and Ken B.,** to name a few more. I hope someday, in another dimension, I will have the opportunity to greet them all again.

Glossary

Biopsy: An examination of living tissue to discover the presence or extent of disease. During a lung biopsy, a very small piece of tissue is taken.

Bronchoscope: A tool usually passed through the nose or mouth used for inspecting the inside of airways (bronchial tubes) of the lungs. Biopsies of the lungs can be performed by bronchoscopy.

Bronchoscopy: An endoscopic technique of visualizing the inside if the airways for diagnostic and therapeutic purposes.

Chest X-ray: An X-ray that produces images of the heart, lungs, airways, and blood vessels, as well as the bones of the spine and chest. A PA/lateral chest X-ray provides a two-dimensional view of the lungs.

Computed tomography (CT) scan: A procedure that uses a combination of X-rays and a computer to create a three-dimensional image of an individual's organs, bones, and other tissues. A CT scan shows more detail than a regular X-ray and is sometimes referred to as a CAT scan.

Echocardiogram: An echo is a graphic outline of the heart's movement.

Exacerbation: An episode of rapid decline or the emergence of more severe symptoms.

Forced expiratory volume (FEV1): The amount of air you can blow out in one second after filling up your lungs with as much air as possible. Measured by a test called spirometry.

Forced vital capacity (FVC): The amount of air you can blow out of your lungs seconds after filling up your lungs with as much air as possible. Measured by a test called spirometry.

Gastroesophageal reflux disease (GERD): A medical condition defined by passage of stomach contents into the esophagus (food pipe) and often into the throat. GERD can cause discomfort ("heartburn" or "acid indigestion") and sometimes injures the lining of the esophagus. Also called acid reflux disease.

Idiopathic: Of unknown cause.

Interstitial lung diseases (ILD): A broad category of over 200 lung diseases that affect the lung interstitium. Typically, ILDs cause inflammation, fibrosis (scarring), or an accumulation of cells in the lung not due to infection or cancer.

Pulmonary: Relating to the lungs.

Pulmonologist: A physician specializing in the lungs.

Radiologist: A physician specializing in using radiology tests (e.g., X-rays) to diagnose illness.

Spirometry: A test that measures the amount of air inhaled and exhaled with each breath.

Abbreviations

ABG: arterial blood gas

CAT: computed axial tomography

CT: computed tomography

EKG: electrocardiogram

FEV: forced expiratory volume

FVC: forced vital capacity

GERD: gastroesophageal reflux disease

HRCT: high-resolution computed tomography

IPF: idiopathic pulmonary fibrosis

LPM: liters per minute

OT: occupational therapist

OSA: obstructive sleep apnea

PT: Physical Therapist

PF: pulmonary fibrosis

PFF: Pulmonary Fibrosis Foundation

PFTs: pulmonary function tests

PFF: Pulmonary Fibrosis Foundation

PR: Pulmonary rehabilitation

ST: Speech Therapist

WBC: White Blood Count

<u>**A final word…**</u>

If you have been on this journey of mine from the start, and by the start, I mean if you have read *New Mountains to Climb* and "*… the kids are still playing nice together in the sandbox*" you have been with me on my journey with this dreaded disease for almost 13 years.

 At this time, I continue to recover extremely well from my second transplant, and I see no reason why this should not continue. With my continued good health, and if I follow my doctors' orders, I see no reason why I will not be around for many years to come.

I leave you with the following saying to think about. I found the following in a magazine, and it sort of sums up this part of my life:

Although I still have pulmonary fibrosis,

I have two scars you can say are proof of my victory

in at least this battle.

I haven't won the war, but I will continue to fight until I do.

Never be ashamed of a scar.

Scars are Proof of victory.

They simply mean you are stronger than whatever tried to hurt you.

Peace and good health to all.…

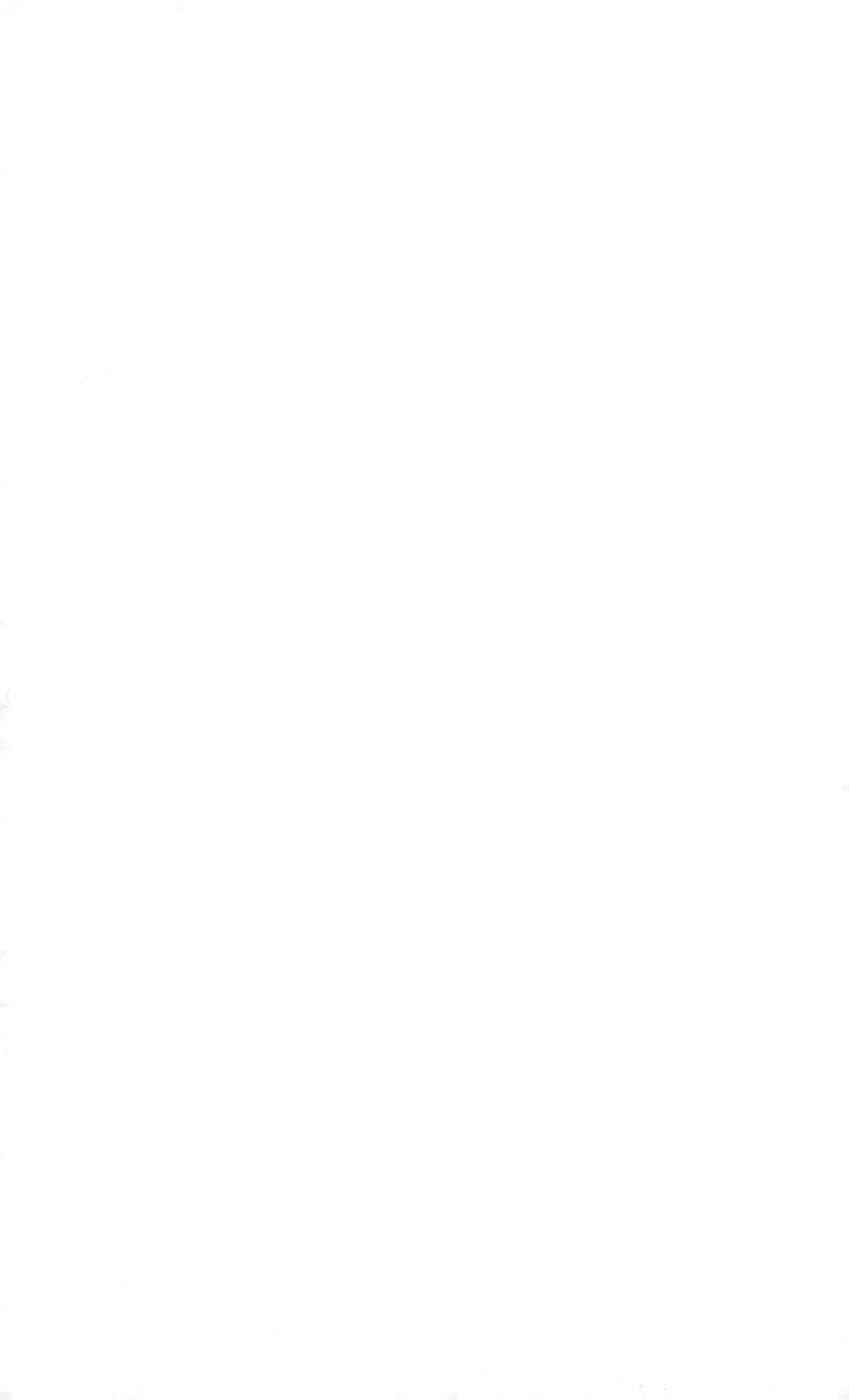